AF698269

MEDICAL PROCEDURES, TESTING AND TECHNOLOGY

# SCREENING TESTS

## PRINCIPLES, ANALYSIS AND BENEFITS

# MEDICAL PROCEDURES, TESTING AND TECHNOLOGY

Additional books in this series can be found on Nova's website under the Series tab.

Additional e-books in this series can be found on Nova's website under the e-book tab.

MEDICAL PROCEDURES, TESTING AND TECHNOLOGY

# SCREENING TESTS

# PRINCIPLES, ANALYSIS AND BENEFITS

MARGUERITE GAUTHIER
EDITOR

*New York*

Copyright © 2013 by Nova Science Publishers, Inc.

**All rights reserved.** No part of this book may be reproduced, stored in a retrieval system or transmitted in any form or by any means: electronic, electrostatic, magnetic, tape, mechanical photocopying, recording or otherwise without the written permission of the Publisher.

For permission to use material from this book please contact us:
Telephone 631-231-7269; Fax 631-231-8175
Web Site: http://www.novapublishers.com

## NOTICE TO THE READER

The Publisher has taken reasonable care in the preparation of this book, but makes no expressed or implied warranty of any kind and assumes no responsibility for any errors or omissions. No liability is assumed for incidental or consequential damages in connection with or arising out of information contained in this book. The Publisher shall not be liable for any special, consequential, or exemplary damages resulting, in whole or in part, from the readers' use of, or reliance upon, this material. Any parts of this book based on government reports are so indicated and copyright is claimed for those parts to the extent applicable to compilations of such works.

Independent verification should be sought for any data, advice or recommendations contained in this book. In addition, no responsibility is assumed by the publisher for any injury and/or damage to persons or property arising from any methods, products, instructions, ideas or otherwise contained in this publication.

This publication is designed to provide accurate and authoritative information with regard to the subject matter covered herein. It is sold with the clear understanding that the Publisher is not engaged in rendering legal or any other professional services. If legal or any other expert assistance is required, the services of a competent person should be sought. FROM A DECLARATION OF PARTICIPANTS JOINTLY ADOPTED BY A COMMITTEE OF THE AMERICAN BAR ASSOCIATION AND A COMMITTEE OF PUBLISHERS.

Additional color graphics may be available in the e-book version of this book.

**Library of Congress Cataloging-in-Publication Data**

ISBN: 978-1-62417-963-1

Library of Congress Control Number: 2012956454

*Published by Nova Science Publishers, Inc. † New York*

# CONTENTS

# PREFACE

In this book, the authors gather and present current research in the study of the principles, analysis and benefits of screening tests. Topics discussed include the development of a screening instrument to detect common mental disorders in long-term sickness absence; a vision screening test in newborns; nailfold capillaroscopy as a basic screening tool in Raynaud's phenomenon; the Profile of Moods Scale to assess six dimensions of mood; the Audio Recorded Cognitive Screen (ARCS) as a flexible and versatile instrument of clinical and research settings.

Chapter 1 – Common Mental Disorders (CMD) are frequent in society in general, and in long-term sickness absence (LSA) in particular. The disorders cause severe suffering for the sick-listed individuals and their relatives, economic burdens on society and challenges for rehabilitation services. CMD are undetected by about 50% in several contexts, e.g. in rehabilitation back to work. The consequence is that the sick-listed individuals with undetected CMD are referred to rehabilitative measures ill-suited for them due to the CMD. Screening is often recommended merely based on statistical summary statistics such as the Area Under the Curve (AUC) in ROC analyses. However, additional issues in regard to the implementation of a screening program need to be considered before making such a decision. These issues refer to the disease which the screening is intended to detect as well as the screening test itself, not to mention the screening program. These issues are addressed by applying the principles for screening on a previous study, the Central Jutland LSA study, which was carried out by the author. The source of the study was a 37 item screening instrument, Common Mental Disorders – Screening Questionnaire (CMD-SQ), which has been validated in primary care. The instrument is composed of items from the validated screening instruments

SCL-SOM, SCL-8, SCL-ANX4, and SCL-DEP6 which derives from SCL-90R along with Whiteley-7 and CAGE. The validation process of screening tests is described with regard to predictive validity, construct validity, sensitivity to change over time, scalability and monotonicity of the tested scales, and the clinical outcomes. The study, presents a statistical method taking the capacity of the psychiatric services into account in deciding at what level the screening instrument should be implemented. The biases of screening are discussed as well. The Central Jutland LSA Study was carried out in a well-defined population of 118,000 individuals in Denmark where all sick-listed individuals were identifiable. The study included individuals just entering LSA which was defined as eight continuous weeks of sickness absence. Over one year 2,414 individuals entered LSA, and, out of the 2,414 individuals, 1,121 individuals participated in the study. The participants were screened for mental disorders by CMD-SQ. By means of a two-phase methodology, 337 individuals participated in a psychiatric examination where Present State Examination was applied as a diagnostic gold standard. The conclusion is that CMD are disorders suitable for screening and a 13 item scale SCL-8AD was found applicable as a screening instrument.

Chapter 2 – The early detection of visual disorders is important in order to minimize the consequences of visual impairment or delayed visual maturation, especially in newborn or preterm children with and without other disorders such as brain injuries or heart disease. The implementation of early intervention programs is essential. Research has provided evidence that certain visual abilities are present from birth. Instruments designed to detect these abilities include those created by Atkinson's and Ricci's teams and the ML-Leonhardt Optotype Battery which assesses visual functions and distinguishes between reflex and perceptive vision. This chapter describes the ML-Leonhardt Optotype Battery and discusses the results obtained in term and preterm newborns with and without injuries. The data indicate that preterm infants with brain lesions showed a delayed pattern of visual functions in alertness, fixation, visual attention and tracking behavior when compared to healthy preterm infants of around 30%. These visual functions can be identified in the first weeks of life. This early period in life is characterized by enormous sensitivity. When a visual disorder is detected, the initiation of visual stimulation enhances the infant's potential for change. A multidisciplinary approach involving neonatologists, ophthalmologists and neurologists is key to early detection.

Chapter 3 – The term "Raynaud's phenomenon" refers to a defined triphasic colour change pattern (white, blue, red) of the skin of the fingers. The initial pallor, which may lead to cyanosis (blue coloration) of the digits, is followed by reactive hyperemia and can be accompanied by numbness, paresthesias and pain. Raynaud's is triggered by exposure to cold, emotional stress and specific drugs. Pathophysiologically it is characterized by an excessive vasoconstrictive response (dominance of vasoconstrisctive over vasodilatory factors) of the small arterioles and the digital arteries. Etiologically it can be classified as primary or secondary, mainly either to systemic sclerosis and related diseases, or to the thoracic outlet syndrome. As such, Raynaud's phenomenon represents an important clinical manifestation of microvascular involvement. Rare cases of paraneoplastic Raynaud's have been described, the pathogenesis of which remains unclarified, has however been most likely attributed to neuroendocrine substances secreted by the tumor. Despite the evolution of the technology involved over the decades, nailfold capillaroscopy remains very simple in principle. The term refers to the non-invasive observation of the nailfold capillary bed. Nailfold capillaroscopy can be performed with basic equipment such as a magnifying lens, an ophthalmoscope, a dermatoscope/ stereomicroscope or a conventional wide field microscope; the nailfold video capillaroscope, however, is the gold standard tool, and provides the technology for the visualization and analysis both of morphological as well as rheological parameters of the skin microvasculature. Qualitative and quantitative microangiopathic parameters that can be recorded and analyzed include, among others, microhemorrhages, plexus morphology, capillary density, and morphologic anomalies of the end row loops. In normal conditions, or in primary Raynaud's, the normal nailfold capillaroscopic pattern shows a regular disposition of the capillary loops along with the nailbed. In subjects suffering from secondary Raynaud's phenomenon, alterations of the capillaroscopic findings should alert the physician of the possibility of a connective tissue disease or other conditions not yet detected. This review aims to outline the major characteristics of the normal nailfold microvascular network and the healthy variations that may be encountered in relation to age, race, employment etc, and highlight its applicability not only as a powerful tool in the screening of a variety of vascular disorders, in particular of autoimmune origin, but also as a potent tool in the follow-up of patients with established microvascular disorders in response to treatment. As microcirculation involvement is attracting increasing interest in chronic vascular diseases such as diabetes mellitus or hypertension, as a prognostic marker for macrovascular disease and target organ involvement, the acquaintance with and application of techniques assessing microvascular compromise gains particular significance. The advantages of capillaroscopy (low cost, uninvasiveness, repeatability, high sensitivity, good specificity and easy interpretation of the results) render this technique a valuable asset for the clinician.

Chapter 4 – The factorial structure of the short form Profile of Moods Scale (POMS; McNair, Lorr, and Droppleman, 1992) was examined based on responses to the scale by 290 adults (122 men and 168 women). The short form POMS is a 30-item scale designed to assess six dimensions of mood: Vigor, Tension, Fatigue, Depression, Confusion, and Anger. The short form of the POMS was derived from the longer 65-item scale which was developed using factor analytic techniques, although this statistical method was not used in the generation of the short form of the scale. Following an analysis of the factorial structure of the short form items, five of the six scales were found to fit the proposed pattern; the exception was for the items measuring Confusion.

Chapter 5 – The ARCS was developed as a medium length cognitive battery that, by virtue of its novel means of administration, can also serve as a screening test. The ARCS includes tests of episodic verbal memory, verbal fluency, language (object naming), visuospatial ability, and attention/executive functioning that are administered via an audio device (e.g. MP3 player, CD player, computer). The patient (or study participant) writes their responses to the questions in a booklet for later scoring. A preamble on the audio provides a clear and simple explanation as to how testing will be conducted. Testing lasts 34 minutes and is unsupervised. Patients who score 18/30 or more on the Mini Mental State Examination are typically able to complete testing with the ARCS. The time-cost to the clinician for obtaining the results is minimal: about two minutes to set the patient up with the audio and response booklet and about 2-4 minutes for scoring into the accompanying excel spreadsheet scoring calculator. The calculator converts raw scores into demographically adjusted scores and also serves as a database. The current chapter reviews our experience with the ARCS, highlighting its flexibility, and discusses its potential use in a range of clinical and research settings.

In: Screening Tests
Editor: Marguerite Gauthier
ISBN: 978-1-62417-963-1
© 2013 Nova Science Publishers, Inc.

*Chapter 1*

# The Development of a Screening Instrument to Detect Common Mental Disorders in Long-Term Sickness Absence

***Hans Joergen Soegaard***
Psychiatric Research Unit West, Regional Psychiatric Services West, Central Region Denmark, Gl. Landevej, Herning, Denmark

## Abstract

Common Mental Disorders (CMD) are frequent in society in general, and in long-term sickness absence (LSA) in particular. The disorders cause severe suffering for the sick-listed individuals and their relatives, economic burdens on society and challenges for rehabilitation services. CMD are undetected by about 50% in several contexts, e.g. in rehabilitation back to work. The consequence is that the sick-listed individuals with undetected CMD are referred to rehabilitative measures ill-suited for them due to the CMD.

Screening is often recommended merely based on statistical summary statistics such as the Area Under the Curve (AUC) in ROC analyses. However, additional issues in regard to the implementation of a screening program need to be considered before making such a decision. These issues refer to the disease which the screening is intended to detect as well as the screening test itself, not to mention the screening program.

These issues are addressed by applying the principles for screening on a previous study, the Central Jutland LSA study, which was carried out by the author.

The source of the study was a 37 item screening instrument, Common Mental Disorders – Screening Questionnaire (CMD-SQ), which has been validated in primary care. The instrument is composed of items from the validated screening instruments SCL-SOM, SCL-8, SCL-ANX4, and SCL-DEP6 which derives from SCL-90R along with Whiteley-7 and CAGE.

The validation process of screening tests is described with regard to predictive validity, construct validity, sensitivity to change over time, scalability and monotonicity of the tested scales, and the clinical outcomes. The study, presents a statistical method taking the capacity of the psychiatric services into account in deciding at what level the screening instrument should be implemented. The biases of screening are discussed as well.

The Central Jutland LSA Study was carried out in a well-defined population of 118,000 individuals in Denmark where all sick-listed individuals were identifiable. The study included individuals just entering LSA which was defined as eight continuous weeks of sickness absence. Over one year 2,414 individuals entered LSA, and, out of the 2,414 individuals, 1,121 individuals participated in the study. The participants were screened for mental disorders by CMD-SQ. By means of a two-phase methodology, 337 individuals participated in a psychiatric examination where Present State Examination was applied as a diagnostic gold standard.

The conclusion is that CMD are disorders suitable for screening and a 13 item scale SCL-8AD was found applicable as a screening instrument.

## INTRODUCTION

The term "Common Mental Disorders" (CMD) refers to the most frequent mental disorders in a population. The most frequent CMD are depression, anxiety, and somatoform disorder. A meta-analysis of population studies have shown the following 12-month prevalence: anxiety disorders 12%, mood disorders 9%, and somatoform disorders 11% [1]. The basis of this chapter is the Central Jutland LSA Study which comprised all incident individuals on LSA. In this study, the same disorders also showed to be the most frequent with the following prevalence: 35% for depression, 15% for anxiety, 7% for somatoform disorder, and 5% for alcohol- and substance abuse [2].

CMD impose suffering and reduced quality of life on the sick-listed individuals and their relatives [3-8]. Depressive disorders significantly influence the outcome of comorbid medical illnesses such as cardiac diseases, diabetes, and cancer [3;9]. Furthermore, the disorders also place economic burdens on society, primarily due to indirect costs in regards to sickness absence, early retirement, and early death [3;8;10-13;13-15]. The burden is increasing as mental health problems in OECD countries now account for a third of all new disability benefit claims on average, and in some countries nearly 50% [16]. The cumulative incidence of sick-listed individuals with CMD on LSA is increasing [17].

The suffering and burden may be more widespread than what appears from official statistics due to the fact that CMD frequently are undetected such as documented in general practice [18-20], in the granting of disability pension [21-23], in non-specialist settings [24;25], among patient populations such as patients with, e.g. chronic musculoskeletal pain [26], and in sick-leave certificates [27;28]. With regard to the undetected CMD, one consequence is that the sick-listed individuals with undetected CMD are referred to rehabilitative measures ill-suited for them, namely due to the CMD. The result is a new defeat and prolongation of the sickness absence period. On this background it seems obvious to implement a screening program for CMD.

Several meta-analyses and reviews regarding screening studies have been carried out for studies of primary care and non-specialist settings [24;25;29;30]. Gilbody et al. [24;25] only found a minimal impact on the detection of mental disorders by screening. However, Hickie et al. [29] concluded that screening increases the detection and diagnosis of depression, and when integrated with a commitment to provide a coordinated and prompt follow-up on diagnosis and treatment, clinical outcomes were improved. Pignone et al. [30] also concluded that screening combined with feedback to the caregivers increased the detection of depressive illness, and, furthermore, reduced the risk of persistent depression. Programs which integrated interventions with quality improvements in clinical systems had stronger effects than programs consisting of feedback alone. The reviews did not address the effect on sickness absence however.

## AIM

With regard to validation of screening instruments, several studies are often limited to the presentation of summary statistics of validity measures for potential screening instruments. However, before a screening program is introduced, several other aspects have to be considered; aspects which apply to: 1) The disease which the screening instrument is intended to screen for, 2) The screening instrument itself, and 3) The screening program. The aim of this chapter is to analyze these aspects in relation to the Central Jutland LSA Study involving validation of potential screening instruments by analysing the following questions [2;31-38]: 1) Are CMD suitable for screening?, 2) Is there a test for detection of CMD which take into account the capacity of psychiatric services to follow up on screening?, and 3) What implications do the analyses entail for a screening program?

# METHODS

## Characteristics of Screening

The activity of screening has a history of more than 100 years. Among other aims, screening has been used by life-insurance companies and employers to evaluate the future health and mortality of policyholders and employee's. However, in this context it is the application of a screening program in improving the health of a population that will be addressed [39;40].

## Definition of Screening

Over time, several definitions of screening have been developed and employed. In the context of this chapter and the Central Jutland LSA study, it is the definition by Eddy [41] that is applied, however, modified. The definition states that screening is the application of a test to detect a potential disease or a condition in an individual who has no known signs or symptoms of that disease or condition [41]. The modification refers to an extension of the definition to include the detection of diseases or conditions that manifest clinical signs or symptoms which are not recognized [39].

## Objectives of Screening

The major objectives of screening are the following [41;42]:

1) Detection of disease at a stage without signs or symptoms and at which stage treatment is more effective than it would be after the patient develops signs or symptoms. Furthermore, the objective is detection of disease with manifest clinical signs or symptoms, however unrecognized.

or

2) Identification of a risk factor that increases the likelihood of developing a disease and where use of this knowledge is used for the prevention or lessening of the disease by modifying the risk factors.

From a primary glance, screening may seem an unequivocally positive activity as the intention of screening is to recognize a disease at an earlier stage with the aim of initiating treatment earlier. This, in turn, is expected to generate a more positive treatment outcome. However, a deeper examination of the activity reveals that screening may be both beneficial and harmful to individuals and society. The implementation of a screening program is a trade-off between these two positions. In order to reach a position where a screening program does more good than harm some principles must be taken into account before the decision to implement a screening program is made. The principles should be considered with regard to the disease, the potential screening test, and the screening program in question. The screening program refers to the entire set-up of the screening procedures in relation to the screened individuals and at an organisational level. The principles were launched by Wilson & Jungner [40] and, with some modifications, the principles are [39;40;42]:

For the disease in question:

1) The disease poses a serious health problem
2) The disease has a high prevalence in the preclinical phase among the population targeted for screening
3) Treatment is beneficial before the development of clinical signs and symptoms as well as of unrecognized clinical cases and an accepted treatment is available
4) The disease has a critical point before which treatment is efficacious
5) The disease has a low incidence of pseudodisease

For the test in question:

6) The test is capable of detecting a high proportion of disease in its preclinical state as well as of clinical manifest but unrecognized disease
7) The test is safe to administer and acceptable to the population
8) The test is reasonable in cost, and it has demonstrated improved health outcomes
9) The test is widely available, as are the interventions that follow a positive result

For the screening program in question:

10) The progam has facilities for diagnosis and treatment available and it has an agreed policy on whom to treat as patients
11) The program is able to implement continuous case-finding for all eligible patients.

A critical point refers to a point in the development of a disease before which treatment is more efficacious than after, e.g. for cancer the development of metastases is a critical point. Pseudodisease refers to a disease that is detected by screening but does not require treatment because it does not progress into symptomatic disease, and it doesn't affect the patients' length of life or quality of life in a significant way. Screening will be ineffective if it reveals substantial pseudodisease.

## Screening for CMD in LSA

The study on which this chapter focuses, the Central Jutland LSA Study [2;31-38], analyses the development of a screening instrument for CMD; consequently, the aim is delimited to the first objective [41;42].

### *Screening Instruments*

With the aim of screening for CMD, several screening instruments have been validated in primary care such as the validation of Common Mental Disorders - Screening Questionnaire (CMD-SQ) [19;43-45], the General Health Questionnaire (GHQ) [46], and its short form, GHQ-12 [47], the Primary Care Evaluation of Mental Disorders (PRIME-MD) [48;49], and the Symptom Driven Diagnostic System for Primary Care (SDDS-PC) [50]. In the Central Jutland LSA Study, it was considered reasonable to apply CMD-SQ because it has been validity tested in primary care in a Danish context, and it is intended for the detection CMD which are the most frequent disorders in both the fields of primary care and LSA [45].

***Study Population of the Central Jutland LSA Study***

The study took place in a well-defined population of approximately 118,000 inhabitants in Denmark. In Denmark, all sick listed individuals are easily identifiable because sickness absence benefits are publicly registered, and, thus, the study was based on comprehensive registers. The eligible study population comprised all 2,414 incident individuals on sickness absence, who had their first day of sickness absence between the 30th of August 2004 and the 29th of August 2005, and who later proceeded into LSA. LSA was defined as a continued sickness absence period exceeding eight weeks. Only the first sickness absence period exceeding eight weeks, within the year that was studied, was included. The following persons were excluded: Persons under 18 years of age at the day when the sickness absence period exceeded eight weeks, persons unable to understand Danish, and persons absent from work due to pregnancy and childbirth.

***Common Mental Disorders – Screening Questionnaire (CMD-SQ)***

CMD-SQ is composed of the following subscales: 1) SCL-SOM (somatic distress) [51], 2) SCL-8 (emotional disorder) [52], 3) SCL-ANX4 (anxiety) [45], and 4) SCL-DEP6 (depression) [45] which are all derived from the Symptom Checklist (SCL-90-R) [51]. Furthermore, it includes 5) Whiteley-7 (Illness conviction and worry) [53] and 6) CAGE (alcohol abuse) [54]. In addition, SCL-ANX4, SCL-8, and SCL-DEP6 were compiled into one subscale mentioned SCL-8AD. The items in SCL-8AD are all derived from the self -report symptom scale SCL-90-R, which in several contexts have shown good validity and reliability [51;55].

CMD-SQ is composed of 37 items, of which only 36 were relevant to the Central Jutland LSA Study. ITEMS 1 to 32 were scored on 5-point Likert where 0 = “no symptoms at all” and 4 = “extremely” within the last 4 weeks before filling in the questionnaire. ITEMS 33 to 36 are dichotomized questions indicating alcohol abuse within the last year. Each of the 32 items in CMD-SQ was dichotomized between 0 and 1 making all items dichotomous resulting in dichotomized component scales (DC-scales) with scores ranging between 0 and the number of items, e.g. in regard to SCL-ANX4 with 4 items between 0 and 4. ITEMS 1-32 were also analyzed by the sum of the scores on the Likert scales, sum-scales (S-scales).

**Table 1. SCL-8AD**

| During the last 4 weeks how mutch were you bothered by: | Not at all | A little | Moderately | Quite a bit | Extremely |
|---|---|---|---|---|---|
| Feeling suddenly scared for no reason? | ☐ | ☐ | ☐ | ☐ | ☐ |
| Nervousness or shakiness inside? | ☐ | ☐ | ☐ | ☐ | ☐ |
| Spells of terror or panic? | ☐ | ☐ | ☐ | ☐ | ☐ |
| You worry too much? | ☐ | ☐ | ☐ | ☐ | ☐ |
| Feeling fearful? | ☐ | ☐ | ☐ | ☐ | ☐ |
| Feeling hopeless about the future? | ☐ | ☐ | ☐ | ☐ | ☐ |
| Feeling everything is an effort? | ☐ | ☐ | ☐ | ☐ | ☐ |
| Feeling blue? | ☐ | ☐ | ☐ | ☐ | ☐ |
| Feelings of worthlessness? | ☐ | ☐ | ☐ | ☐ | ☐ |
| Thoughts of ending your life? | ☐ | ☐ | ☐ | ☐ | ☐ |
| Feelings of being trapped or caught? | ☐ | ☐ | ☐ | ☐ | ☐ |
| Feelings of being trapped or caught? | ☐ | ☐ | ☐ | ☐ | ☐ |
| Blaming yourself for things? | ☐ | ☐ | ☐ | ☐ | ☐ |

However, CAGE was not included in the study. Table 1 shows SCL-8AD. The score of the DC-scale is represented by the number of scores right to the highlighted line and the score of the S-scale by the sum of scores.

The DC-scales are symptom scales indicating the number of symptoms, no matter the severity. For a DC-scale with n items n+2 tests were defined, e.g. for SCL-8 consisting of eight items, a test was defined for each cut-point from 0/1 to 7/8 plus the two end-points.

A test was considered positive if the score was at the cut-point or higher, e.g. if a test was considered positive by the cut-point 4/5, the test was positive for a score of 5 or higher and negative for a score of 4 and below. The same was carried out for the S-scales.

Information about the sick-leave diagnoses were gathered from discharge records and other medical documents from the rehabilitation services, and they were coded by the investigator according to the ICPC classification [56].

## RESULTS

The principles of screening [1-11] mentioned on page 7-8 are in the following analyzed with regard to CMD.

### 1. CMD Pose a Serious Health Problem

It is well documented that individuals affected by CMD as well as the relatives of individuals with CMD experience an increased level of psychological distress and have a seriously decreased quality of life [3-7;57-59].

Moreover, depression is associated with an increased risk of suicide [60]. The disorders furthermore pose an increased risk of comorbid disorders such as cardiac diseases and diabetes [3;9;61] which also is the case for children of individuals with depression [58]. In addition, somatic/psychiatric comorbidity increases the suffering and burden [62]. Finally, depression is associated with an increased risk of developing cognitive impairment and dementia [63;64;64-71].

## 2. CMD Have a High Prevalence among the Population Targeted for Screening

The criterion that treatment of a disorder should be beneficial before the development of clinical signs or symptoms does not really apply to CMD according to the original definition. This is due to the fact that CMD are syndrome diagnoses which means that the diagnostic criteria are based on the appearance of definite symptoms within a definite period of time according to the diagnostic classification systems ICD-10 [72] and DSM-IV [73]. In theory, the disorders don't exist before these criteria are met. However, it is reasonable to talk about subclinical states, and even at a subclinical level, the disorders are associated with psychological distress and reduced quality of life [74-76]. CMD usually develop gradually and the disorders are often preceded by stressful life events caused by, e.g. a stressful working environment or stress in other areas of the individuals' lives. In the beginning, the symptoms often are of a somatic nature, such as pain in the musculoskeletal system, gastrointestinal symptoms, cardiovascular symptoms, headache, and tiredness. Due to the somatic nature of the symptoms, focus is, thus, on somatic disorders and the development of psychological symptoms is not recognized immediately.

With regard to preclinical symptoms or signs, no tests are available for use in a clinical context. However, there is growing evidence that the emergence of depression is preceded by an increased activity in the hypothalamic-pituitary axis [77;78].

With regard to the extension of the definition of screening to include undetected diseases that manifest clinical symptoms and signs, the criterion can be applied for CMD due to the fact that CMD are frequently undetected in LSA [2] as well as in other populations [18-28;79]. With reference to LSA, 23% of all individuals have an undetected mental disorder [31;33].

## 3. Treatment of CMD is Beneficial Before the Development of Clinical Signs and Symptoms as well as of Unrecognized Clinical Cases and an Accepted Treatment is Available

It is documented that early treatment with antidepressant medication or psychological therapies reduces the development of recurrences or chronic development of the CMD [80-87], suicidal risk [60;88;89] and development of cognitive impairment and dementia [63;64;64-71]. This is also of relevance for subclinical cases [74-76]. Antidepressant medication and psychological therapies are widely accepted according to the guidelines for treatment [90-92].

## 4. CMD Have a Critical Point before Which Treatment Is Efficacious

With regard to the existence of a critical point, no biological points are applicable in a clinical context at this moment. However, a study of individuals on LSA with job stress-induced depression showed that individuals on LSA had an attenuated response on the dex-RCH test. It remains to be established, however, if this impairment is the result of prolonged stress exposure or a pre-existing susceptibility factor [78]. The development of reduced volumes of hippocampus and the prefrontal cortex before the initiation of treatment must also be considered as a critical point as the reduced volumes are supposed to be a consequence of the elevated level of glucocorticoids in prolonged stress [93].

On a psychological and social level there are more critical points due to the fact that CMD cause new stressors such as social isolation and sickness absence, which in the long run causes a threat to the individuals' socio-economic situation. The latter situation is certainly true if there are limitations as to how long sickness absence benefits are paid. The stressors are sustained which again contributes to the burden on the hypothalamic-pituitary axis and a vicious circle is established.

## 5. CMD Have a Low Incidence of Pseudodisease

Pseudodisease refers to the situation where a screening test identifies individuals with a disease which is of no importance to the individuals' length of life or quality of life but who, based on the screening result, go through a diagnostic procedure or treatment which is potentially harmful or burdensome to the individual. With regard to pseudodiseases resembling CMD, there is no clear-cut pseudodisease. However, the disorders constitute a continuum with regard to number, severity, and duration of symptoms. Consequently, screening for CMD will probably result in positive tests of some individuals for whom the condition would have disappeared without treatment. The consequence of a positive screening test for individuals with a pseudodisease is that the individuals go through an unnecessary psychiatric examination. However, neither the screening nor the diagnostic examination is harmful to the individual but the psychiatric examination imposes a burden on the individual and on the psychiatric services. Furthermore, no individuals commence a potential harmful treatment without a psychiatric examination.

## 6. The Test is Capable of Detecting a High Proportion of Disease in its Preclinical State as Well as of Clinical Manifest But Unrecognized Disease

Screening for CMD is based on the recognition of psychological symptoms according to the diagnostic classification systems ICD-10 [72] and DSM-IV [73]. The screening is most often carried out by the individual's self rating on symptom scales of psychological distress. This was the case in the Central Jutland LSA study with regard to CMD-SQ. A summary of the validity testing is presented in the following psychometric analyses [32;34;37].

***Predictive Validity***

I can be discussed whether we are dealing with predictive validity or concurrent validity as both are generally measured as correlations between a test and some criterion measure. Due to the fact that both validities are generally measured as correlations between a test and a defined criterion measure, it is a matter of discussion whether or not the study deals with predictive or concurrent validity. In concurrent validity testing, the test is administered at the same time as information about the criterion is collected, whereas in predictive validity testing, the criterion is collected at a later point in time [94]. In the Central Jutland LSA study 90% of the screening results were collected within two weeks of the individuals entering LSA. The criterion was defined as the diagnostic results of the psychiatric examination which was collected as soon as possible after entering LSA. However, there was a delay before a psychiatric examination could be carried out. The diagnostic results were collected for 10% within 20 days, 50% within 29 days, and 90% within 45 days. The longest delay was 73 days.

The criterion was established by a diagnostic interview by a psychiatrist who applied SCAN, version 2.1, program version 1.0.4.6, Present State Examination (PSE) as gold standard, period Present Episode. The outcome was ICD-10 diagnoses [72;95].

In psychometrics, testing of predictive validity involves testing of each of the tests embedded in a symptom scale, e.g. SCL-8AD is a 13-point scale which means that each of the tests defined by the cut-points from 0/1 to 12/13 should be tested.

Table 2 shows the definition of the outcome probabilities which are used in predictive validity testing. The essential parameters are: 1) the sensitivity (SE) which indicates the proportion of individuals with a positive test among the individuals who have a disorder. 2) The specificity (SP) which indicates the proportion of individuals with a negative test among the individuals without a disorder. SP is often transformed into 1-SP which is called the false alarm rate. 3) The level of a test, Q, which indicates the random possibility of a positive test, meaning the chance that a subject picked at random from the examined population is test-positive, and 4) The prevalence of the disorder, P.

The other statistical measures in Table 2 are based on these measures. A frequently used method in predictive validity testing is ROC analyses. Figure 1 shows a ROC curve where SE is plotted against 1-SP of SCL-8AD tested for any mental disorder [96]. The analysis shows that when SE goes up, 1-SP also goes up. One measure in ROC analysis is the Area Under Curve (AUC). The value of AUC refers to the area under the curve, and it ranges between 0 and 1. Values near 0.5 indicate no predictive power, whereas values near 1 indicate excellent power. This is also the case for values near 0, however, the prediction is opposite which means that it is a negative test that predicts a disorder. The values of interest are values above 0.5, and they are interpreted as follows: 0.90-1.00 excellent, 0.80-0.90 good, 0.70-0.80 fair, 0.60-0.70 poor, and 0.50-0.60 fail [97]. The AUC refers to a test of all the embedded tests in a symptom scale. However, this measure doesn't indicate which cut-point is optimal. Binary ROC analyses are more informative as this method indicates the AUC for each of the embedded tests in a scale. In Table 2, this is shown for the cut-points 5/6, 6/7, and 7/8 of SCL-8AD.

ROC curves are two-dimensional graphs in which the true-positive rate is plotted on the Y-axis and the false positive rate on the X-axis. A negative quality of ROC analyses is that true positives and true negatives may evolve by chance which is corrected for in QROC analyses [96]. In QROC analyses the decisive measure is κ(r,0) where r is a factor ranging between 0 and 1. The higher r, the higher priority is given to the SE in the analyses. In the Central Jutland LSA study κ(0.5,0) was chosen which indicate equal priority to SE and SP. Values under 0 indicate less than chance agreement, 0.01-0.20 slight agreement, 0.21-0.40 fair agreement, 0.41-0.60 moderate agreement, 0.61-0.80

substantial agreement, and 0.81-0.99 almost perfect agreement in the prediction of a disorder [98].

**Table 2. Decisive measures in studies of predictive validity**

| | | Test reult | | |
|---|---|---|---|---|
| | | + | - | |
| Diagnosis | + | TP | FN | P |
| | - | FP | TN | P'=1 - P |
| | | Q | Q'=1 - Q | 1 |

TP = true positive FN = false negative

FP = False positive TN = true negative

Prevalence = P = TP + FN

Level of a Positive Test = Q = TP + FP

Level of a Negative Test = Q′= 1-Q = FN + TN

Efficiency = TP + TN

Sensitivity = SE = TP/P

Specificity = SP = TN/(1-P)

Predictive value of positive test = PVP = TP/Q

Predictive value of negative test = PVN = TN/Q'

$\kappa(1.0,0) = (SE - Q)/Q' = (Q'P - FN)/(Q'P)$

$\kappa(0.0,0) = (SP - Q')/Q = (QP' - FP)/(QP')$

$\kappa(r,0) = (P * Q' * r * \kappa(1,0) + P' * Q * r' * \kappa(0,0)) / (P * Q' * r + P' * Q * r')$

$\kappa(0.5,0) = (PQ'\kappa(1.0,0) + P'Q\kappa(0.0,0))/(PQ' + P'Q)$

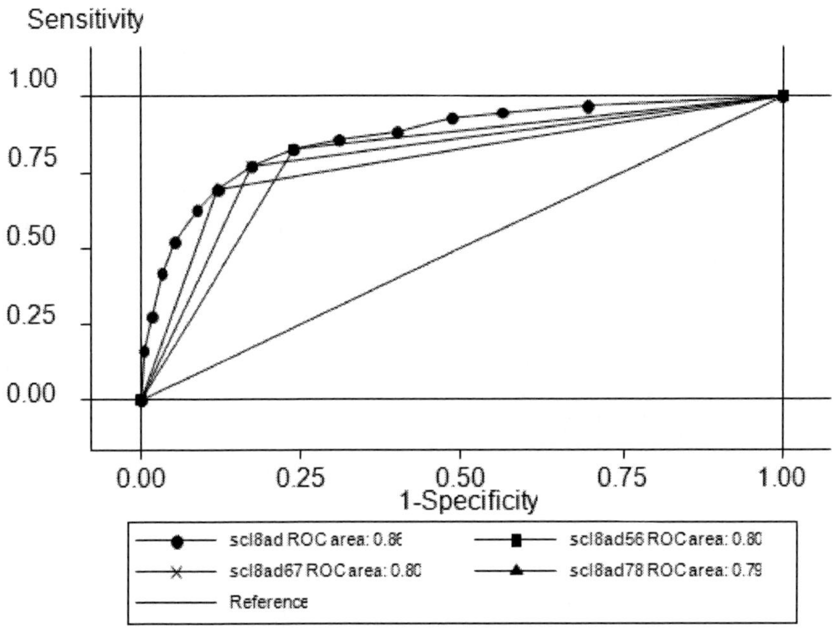


Figure 1. ROC curves of SCL-8AD, SCL-8AD, cut5/6, SCL-8AD, cut6/7, and SCL-8AD, cut7/8 in the detection of any mental disorder.

### *Analyses of the Subscales in CMD-SQ*

The predictive validity were analysed for the subscales of CMD-SQ and the sick-leave diagnoses. Analyses were carried out for both the DC-scales and the S-scales, but due to the fact the DC-scales performed better than the S-scales, only results for the DC-scales are presented. The analyses were carried out for different subgroups but only results for all individuals on LSA are presented. Finally, the analyses were carried out with regard to any psychiatric diagnosis, CMD, any depression, any anxiety, and any somatoform disorder. Any psychiatric diagnosis refers to any psychiatric diagnosis detected by the diagnostic examination. The methods are described in more detail elsewhere [37].

### *Results of the Predictive Analyses*

Based on several analyses the main results are presented in Fiugre 4. The measure κ(0.5,0) was just a little better for the optimal cut-point of SCL-8AD than for the sick-leave diagnoses in all diagnostic groups. The same results are reflected in the Binary AUCs. Furthermore, it appears that SCL-8AD performs on the same level or slightly better than SCL-8, SCL-DEP6, and SCL-ANX4 in the detection of depression and anxiety. SCL-8AD also performs well in the prediction of any mental disorder and CMD, which is due to the fact that these groups primarily are composed of individuals with depression or anxiety which appear from the prevalence shown in Table 3.

**Table 3. Main predictive results indicating, disorder, symptom scale, optimal cut-point, prevalence, level of a positive test Q, sensitivity SE, specificity SP, Binary AUC and κ(0.5,0)**

| Diagnosis/ test | Optimal cut-point | P % | Q % | SE % | SP % | Binary AUC | κ(0.5,0) |
|---|---|---|---|---|---|---|---|
| **Any mental disorder** | | | | | | | |
| Sick-leave diagnosis | - | 48 | 27 | 56 | 99 | 0.78 | 0.59 |
| SCL-SOM | 7/8 | | 32 | 47 | 82 | 0.64 | 0.29 |
| Whiteley-7 | 4/5 | | 33 | 47 | 80 | 0.64 | 0.27 |
| SCL-ANX4 | 1/2 | | 52 | 82 | 77 | 0.80 | 0.59 |
| SCL-8 | 5/6 | | 38 | 66 | 88 | 0.77 | 0.55 |
| SCL-DEP6 | 2/3 | | 47 | 78 | 82 | 0.80 | 0.59 |
| SCL-8AD | 5/6 | | 50 | 81 | 80 | 0.81 | 0.61 |
| **Common Mental Disorders** | | | | | | | |
| Sick-leave diagnosis | - | 44 | 27 | 57 | 96 | 0.77 | 0.56 |
| SCL-SOM | 7/8 | | 32 | 49 | 81 | 0.65 | 0.31 |
| Whiteley-7 | 5/6 | | 22 | 34 | 88 | 0.61 | 0.24 |
| SCL-ANX4 | 1/2 | | 52 | 83 | 73 | 0.78 | 0.55 |
| SCL-8 | 5/6 | | 38 | 69 | 86 | 0.77 | 0.56 |
| SCL-DEP6 | 2/3 | | 47 | 79 | 78 | 0.79 | 0.57 |
| SCL-8AD | 5/6 | | 50 | 89 | 74 | 0.80 | 0.61 |
| **Depression** | | | | | | | |
| Sick-leave diagnosis | | 35 | 27 | 60 | 91 | 0.76 | 0.53 |
| SCL-SOM | 7/8 | | 32 | 51 | 78 | 0.65 | 0.30 |
| Whiteley-7 | 5/6 | | 22 | 36 | 86 | 0.61 | 0.24 |
| SCL-ANX4 | 1/2 | | 52 | 87 | 67 | 0.77 | 0.49 |
| SCL-8 | 5/6 | | 38 | 75 | 82 | 0.78 | 0.55 |
| SCL-DEP6 | 3/4 | | 34 | 70 | 86 | 0.78 | 0.57 |
| SCL-8AD | 6/7 | | 43 | 83 | 79 | 0.80 | 0.58 |
| **Anxiety** | | | | | | | |

| Diagnosis/ test | Optimal cut-point | P % | Q % | SE % | SP % | Binary AUC | κ(0.5,0) |
|---|---|---|---|---|---|---|---|
| Sick-leave diagnosis | - | 15 | 27 | 70 | 80 | 0.75 | 0.37 |
| SCL-SOM | 9/10 | | 13 | 38 | 91 | 0.65 | 0.30 |
| Whiteley-7 | 5/6 | | 22 | 39 | 81 | 0.60 | 0.17 |
| SCL-ANX4 | 3/4 | | 21 | 56 | 85 | 0.70 | 0.35 |
| SCL-8 | 6/7 | | 18 | 47 | 87 | 0.72 | 0.32 |
| SCL-DEP6 | 3/4 | | 34 | 69 | 72 | 0.71 | 0.27 |
| SCL-8AD | 10/11 | | 21 | 59 | 86 | 0.72 | 0.39 |
| **Somatoform disorder** | | | | | | | |
| Sick-leave diagnosis | - | 7 | 27 | 13 | 74 | 0.43 | 0.00 |
| SCL-SOM | 10/11 | | 8 | 20 | 93 | 0.56 | 0.11 |
| Whiteley-7 | 6/7 | | 13 | 28 | 88 | 0.58 | 0.11 |
| SCL-ANX4 | 2/3 | | 35 | 49 | 66 | 0.57 | 0.05 |
| SCL-8 | 6/7 | | 29 | 46 | 72 | 0.58 | 0.06 |
| SCL-DEP6 | 2/3 | | 47 | 71 | 55 | 0.58 | 0.07 |
| SCL-8AD | 8/9 | | 33 | 54 | 69 | 0.62 | 0.09 |

When it comes to the subscales SCL-SOM and Whiteley-7, detection performance was slight in all diagnostic groups. This was to be expected except for somatoform disorder for which diagnostic group the scales are intended. However, the subscales performed worse in the detection of somatoform disorders than in the detection of disorders in the other diagnostic groups. Indeed, all scales with regard to the detection of somatoform disorder showed only slight values of κ(0.5,0).

Figure 2 shows a plot of SE and 1-SP against Q for SCL-8AD, SCL-8, SCL-ANX4, and SCL-DEP6 for detection of any mental disorder. The cut-points are indicated as marks on the curves. However, it is necessary to count to find a specific cut-point, decreasing cut-point with increasing Q. All tests analyzed are for the same diagnostic group, making the analyses independent of the prevalence of the disorder. The figure shows that SE is higher for SCL-8AD than for any of the other scales, except at Q about 0.5. The SE-curves for SCL-8 and SCL-DEP6 are nearly superimposed, whereas the curve for SCL-ANX4 is lower. The false alarm rate, 1-SP, appears from the figure. The curves are superimposed, except for a higher curve for SCL-ANX4. The analyses indicate that SCL-8AD performs superior in the whole range of Q.

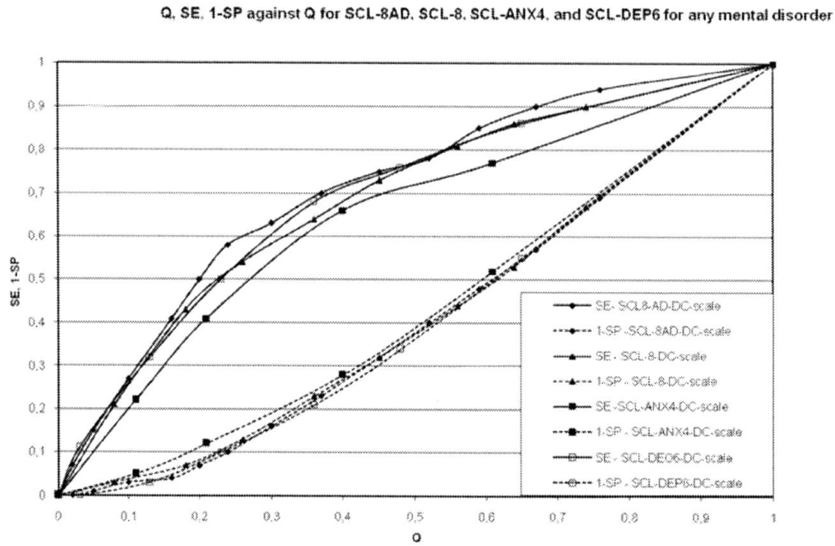


Figure 2. Q, SE, 1-SP against Q for SCL-8AD, SCL-8, SCL-ANX4, and SCL-DEP6 for any mental disorder.

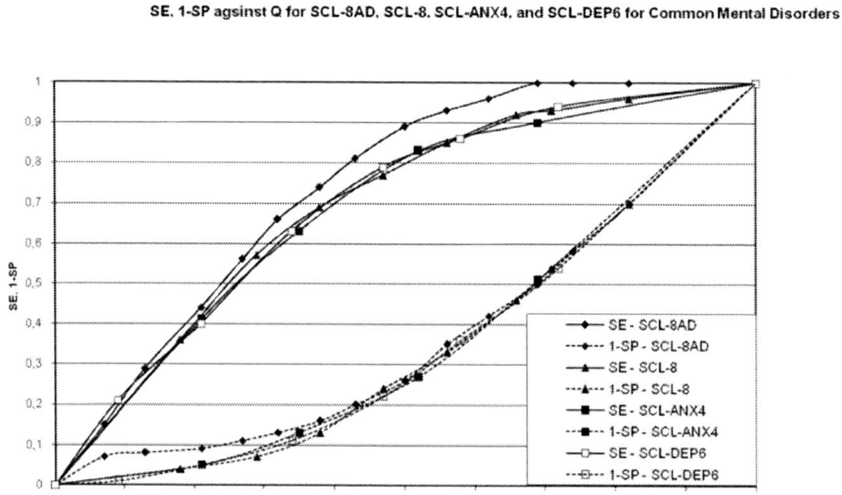


Figure 3. Q, SE, 1-SP against Q for SCL-8AD, SCL-8, SCL-ANX4, and SCL-DEP6 for Common Mental Disorders.

Figure 3 shows a similar plot of SE and 1-SP against Q for SCL-8AD, SCL-8, SCL-ANX4, and SCL-DEP6 in the detection of CMD. It is clear that SCL-8AD performs better than the other scales, and this trend increased as Q increased. Some of the differences are small for which reason the differences may have occurred by chance.

### *Scalability and Monotonicity*

Screening for CMD involves screening for three disorders which may be burdensome in a clinical context because three different symptom scales, one scale for each disorder, have to be applied. However, based on the ROC analyses and QROC analyses mentioned above, it seemed reasonable to apply SCL-8AD in screening for all CMD. The question might be, however, if the 13 items in SCL-8AD screen for the same dimension, and if it is reasonably added up to a score of the positive scored items. Is it reasonable to suspect that even though the disorders are different in appearance they show a common dimension of psychological distress detectable by the symptom scales? These issues were studied by analysing the scalability and the monotonicity (the probability of answering positively to an item step is a non-decreasing function of the latent trait value) of the scales by using non-parametric item response theory as developed by Mokken [34;99]. The monotonicity of a scale is indicated by a Loevinger H coefficient where: $< 0.3$ is unacceptable, 0.3-0.4 is acceptable but weak, 0.4-0.5 is medium and $\geq 0.5$ is strong [99]. Among the examined subscales all subscales, except SCL-SOM, showed Loevinger H coefficients higher than 0.5. In addition, Mokken analyses exclude items in a symptom scale which has an Loevinger H-coefficient below 0.3, so items that constitute another dimension are excluded. The analyses clearly indicated that no items were excluded for SCL-8AD and the Loevinger H was 0.65 signalling that it was safe to consider all items in SCL-8AD as measuring the same dimension. The result is supported by a Danish validation study in a community sample where the 63 non-psychotic items of SCL-90 and SCL-92R appeared to reflect one broad dimension of psychological distress [100].

### *Discriminant Validity, Convergent Validity, and Sensitivity to Change Over Time*

The *discriminant validity* of a scale refers to a low correlation with external references, where a low correlation is expected, and *convergent validity* is high correlation with external references, where a high correlation is expected. *Sensitivity to change* indicates with reference to external references whether the score of a symptom scale reflects changes in the severity of the disorder over time. The S-subscales of CMD-SQ were in the Central Jutland LSA study analysed with regard to discriminant validity, convergent validity, and sensitivity to change over time with external references of SF-36 [34;101;102]. The analyses showed that SCL-8AD had good discriminant and convergent validity, and as for sensitivity to change the results were good as well. These analyses do not relate directly to screening. However, the good psychometric properties of these measuring units indicate that SCL-8AD in addition to screening can be applied in the differentiation of the severity of a condition and in measuring the change of the condition over time in the follow up of patients.

## 7. The Test Is Safe to Administer and Acceptable to the Population

In a screening situation, the individual being tested fills out a questionnaire, which must not in any sense constitute a threat to the individuals' health or safety.

Given that the result of the screening questionnaire is positive, the individual being tested must undergo further psychiatric examinations. A psychiatric examination poses burdens to the individuals and the psychiatric service, however, it does not pose a physical or mental threat to the health of the individual. Furthermore, a decision to start treatment will not be based on a screening result but a clinical examination.

## 8. The Test is Reasonable in Cost and it Has Demonstrated Improved Health Outcomes

The evaluation of a screening program involves an evaluation of: 1) whether or not a screening program is financially viable and efficient, and 2) whether or not the screened individuals show a positive health outcome. In this respect, the Central Jutland LSA study involved a randomized controlled trial which examined the rate of return to work [35] and the effect on psychological distress and quality of life [38]. The intervention was: 1) a psychiatric examination applying a standardized diagnostic gold standard, PSE [103], and 2) feedback to the individuals, general practitioners, and the rehabilitation services with regard to proposed treatment and rehabilitative measures. In regard to cost, the study was not a randomized trial of whether or not screening itself was efficacious but of the efficacy of a psychiatric examination as the randomisation took place after screening.

Overall the intervention showed no significant change in the rate of return to work. In fact, the rate of return to work decreased in the intervention group for the 26% of individuals sick-listed with a psychiatric sick-leave diagnosis. The major explanation of this was that this group of individuals had been mentally ill for some time, but the majority was not referred to psychiatric services leaving them without a specific treatment plan. The psychiatric examinations proposed treatment plans which took some time to establish and the rehabilitative services waited for effect before it was decided if the individuals were ready to return to work.

When it comes to the individuals who were sick-listed without a psychiatric sick-leave diagnosis, however, the study revealed that 30% of them had a psychiatric diagnosis [31]. For this subgroup, the rate of return to work was equal for the intervention group and control group.

However, for the subgroup of individuals sick-listed without a psychiatric sick-leave diagnosis from full time employment, the hazard rate ratio in the time to event analyses were significantly higher (1.31) for return to work in the intervention group. This corresponded to the mean duration of sickness absence being reduced by 65 days in the intervention group. This subgroup constituted 52% of all individuals on LSA; a number of individuals in regard to whom it may be beyond of the capacity of the psychiatric services to offer a psychiatric examination. However, when screening with SCL-8AD DC at cut-point 6/7, the proportion with a positive test constituted 15% of all individuals on LSA which is probably within the capacity of the services. For individuals who met these criteria, the mean reduction in sickness absence days was 132 days in the intervention group. A calculation taking the expenses of sickness benefits and the expenses of carrying out a psychiatric examination into account showed that the savings in sickness absence would be about 3 million € per 100,000 inhabitants per year.

However, the study does not constitute a cost-utility analysis which takes into account the expenses of an increased burden of treatment and measures for quality of life. This has been done by Valenstein et al. [104] in North American primary care. This study found that annual and periodic screening for depression cost more than $50,000/QALY, whereas one-time screening was cost-effective. A cost-utility analysis should also include the costs to establish and run an efficient screening program.

When it comes to the effect on psychological distress and quality of life, the overall effect for individuals sick-listed with a psychiatric sick-leave diagnosis in the intervention group did not result in significant effects. For individuals sick-listed without a psychiatric diagnosis, there were significant effects for all subscales in CMD-SQ, although the effect sizes were small, ranging between 0.20 and 0.28. This was also the case for some of the subscales in SF-36: Bodily Pain, General Health, Role Emotional, Mental Health, and Mental Component Summary showing significant effect sizes between 0.17 and 0.21. Regarding differential effects, one major tendency appeared for individuals sick-listed from full-time work showing significantly positive effects in five subscales in SF36: Physical Function, Role Physical, Bodily Pain, Vitality, and Physical Component Summary with effect sizes between 0.21 and 0.31. The effect sizes were small. However, in the interpretation it is relevant to take into account that the effect sizes were based on the mean effect sizes for subgroups where only about 30% of the individuals were affected with a mental disorder.

## 9. The Test Is Widely Available, As Are the Interventions that Follow a Positive Result

A symptom scale is usually readily available. This is also is the case for SCL-8AD. SCL-8AD is a self-report scale of 13 items and it doesn't take very long to complete the test. The costs with regard to copyright for use of the items which originate from SCL-90 and SCL-90R are low [105;106]. The availability of interventions that follow a positive result is discussed in relation to the predictive validity of the test.

## 10. The Program Has Facilities for Diagnosis and Treatment Available and it Has an Agreed Policy on Whom to Treat as Patients

The establishment and running of a screening program was not the major scope of this chapter. However, the analyses presented in this chapter are preconditions to implementing a screening program. The implementation of a screening program among other issues also involves the establishment a policy for screening, the establishment of an organisation, leadership of the program, and quality assurance of the program which is thoroughly described elsewhere [39;40]. However, the study shows some implications of relevance in regard to these issues.

These issues were discussed in relation to the analyses of the plots of SE and 1-SP against Q in the decision of what level of a test to be used. The chosen level of a test is a trade-off between the number of detected individuals and the psychiatric services' capacity to carry out psychiatric examinations. Furthermore, in this trade-off, it has to be taken into consideration that a screening program will detect more patients who need treatment which is a cost beyond the costs for screening and diagnostics. In the Central Jutland LSA study, the treatment was carried out by the general practitioners on the basis of advice given from the psychiatric examination. However, it is known to the author that some individuals were referred to the psychiatric services on the grounds of the psychiatric examination. Consequently, it is essential prior to implementation of a screening program to have an agreed upon policy of the specific health services that are to follow up on a positive test and diagnosis. These could be the psychiatric services, general practitioners or psychologists in private practice.

## 11. The Program Is Able to Implement Continuous Case-Finding for All Eligible Patients

It is of importance that a screening program is able to carry out screening and follow up on all individuals who screen positive. In the setting of the Central Jutland LSA study, this meant following up on the entire group of eligible individuals. In a Danish context, it is uncomplicated to identify all individuals on LSA because sickness benefits are paid out via public registers comprising all individuals on LSA. This may be different in other countries where payment of sickness benefits is based on private insurance or insurance through one's workplace.

However, even in a context where all individuals can be identified, some individuals may be lost to screening because screening is dependent on informed consent from the individuals. In this regard the Central Jutland LSA study, only about half of the eligible individuals participated. The reason may that the study was sent out from a psychiatric department which in itself might leave potential participants feeling stigmatized by a mental disorder. The response from numerous individuals was that they felt stigmatized and associated with a psychiatric disorder by being presented with the screening instrument or they felt that the screening instrument was of no significance to them. To overcome the stigmatisation affected with mental disorders is a matter of information on a societal level but also on an individual level by the officers that administer the screening. It is also a matter for these officers to convince individuals that screening is a measure which is helpful in the clarification of the psychological distress, the individuals may feel, even though they do not regard themselves as mentally ill. In addition, even if screening results in a positive test, and even if a mental disorder is documented at the psychiatric examination, there may still be obstacles by the diseased individuals in accepting to be affected by a mental disorder and accepting initiation of treatment. The issue is related to the "Healthy screenee effect" bias which is discussed later.

Another matter is *when* and *where* it would be appropriate and suitable to carry out the screening. The screening itself should be applied at the time *when* the sick-listed individuals enter LSA. The validity tests in the Central Jutland LSA study were carried out under these conditions. However, if the conditions change, the results of the validity tests may change as well.

With regard to *where,* this decision may differ from country to country due to the fact that rehabilitation back to work is organized quite dissimilarly across countries. General practice would seem an obvious place. However, in Denmark, where the Central Jutland study was carried out, sick-listed individuals are not required to seek out their general practitioner if the rehabilitation services find the reason for sickness absence clarified in other ways. However, the sick-listed individuals are required to be in contact with their rehabilitation officers before entering LSA. Consequently, it is the logical choice in Denmark to establish screening in this context. As mentioned, this differs from country to country and a screening program ought to be applied in a context where all sick-listed individuals are met by officials. Otherwise, an organisation where all sick-listed are registered must be established and this is likely to impose further costs to such a program. It is a necessity that the rehabilitation officers or others in charge of the screening program are educated in the principles of screening, the benefits of screening, information about a positive screening result not necessarily being equal to a diagnosis, and that sick-listed individuals are not stigmatized by screening.

# DISCUSSION

## Are CMD Suitable for Screening?

CMD are serious and the Central Jutland LSA study showed that several clinical cases are undetected. Treatment of the disorders at an early stage prevents CMD from progressing into a more serious state. It is considered essential to initiate treatment before the development of psychosocial critical points such as sickness absence. No pseuodisease is known.

## Is There a Test for the Detection of CMD Which Take into Consideration the Capacity of Psychiatric Services to Follow Up on Screening?

The analyses in the Central Jutland LSA study showed that SCL-8AD has good properties in detecting CMD. It is safe to administer, its application demonstrated improved health and financial outcomes for individuals who were sick-listed without a psychiatric sick-leave diagnosis, and it is widely available.

The used plots of SE and 1-SP against Q made it possible to adapt the level of a positive test to the capacity of psychiatric services to follow up on a positive screening result.

Delimiting screening to a subgroup of individuals sick-listed without a psychiatric diagnosis from fulltime work made SCL-8AD financially viable. However, economic analyses depend on the costs and subpopulations drawn into account. The study in this chapter does not constitute a cost-utility analysis taking expenses of an increased burden of treatment and measures of quality of life into account. This has been done by Valenstein et al. [104] in American primary care. The study found that annual and periodic screening for depression cost more than $50,000/QALY, whereas one-time screening was cost-effective. With regard to the subpopulation of LSA which are sick-listed without a sick-leave diagnosis and from full time work, it is supposed that the individuals had a newly developed CMD, and, consequently, the majority of the group could be treated by their general practitioners based on the feedback given in the intervention. If this is so, the economic challenges with regard to treatment may even decrease as it is likely to presume that the individuals, even though their mental illness was undetected, would still consult their general practitioner due to their psychological distress. However, this hypothesis needs an economic evaluation on a superior level applying information from public registers with regard to socio-demographic characteristics, admissions to hospitals, emergency rooms and outpatient clinics, redeemed prescriptions on psychoactive drugs, and registers for unemployment benefits, sickness absence benefits and other public benefits [107-110].

The validation of screening instruments are often based on statistical measures such as AUC in ROC analyses and κ(r,0) in QROC analyses. However, The Central Jutland Study illustrated a limited value of these measures when the capacity of services to follow up on a positive screening test is taken into consideration. Based on AUC in ROC analyses and κ(r,0) in QROC analyses, it seemed that the sick-leave diagnosis was equally as good as SCL-8AD at cut-point 5/6. However, the SEs were much lower for the sick-leave diagnosis than for SCL-8AD, except for anxiety. In contrast, the SPs were much higher for the sick-leave diagnosis than for SCL-8AD, and there was an increasing level of positive tests, Q, with increasing SE. In a clinical context, the situation is a trade-off between a high SE and a high SP. In this respect, the level of a test is of interest as it indicates the proportion of the population for whom a diagnostic examination should be offered which again is of relevance in regard to the capacity of the psychiatric services to follow up on screening. The summary statistics AUC and κ(0.5,0) are not of relevance until it is decided at which level of a positive test a screening program should be applied.

If a screening program is intended for a very serious disorder, the clinical situation may be that the diagnostic services allocate plenty of resources to detect the disorder and then it is advisable to choose a low cut-point with a high SE. If the diagnostic services, on the other hand, have limited resources it makes sense to decide on a specific fraction of the population, on which the services are capable of doing examinations. By employing the plots of SE and 1-SP against Q, it appears that for the best test pointed out by the QROC analyses, the SCL-8AD – DC-scale at cut-point 5/6, the level of a positive test was 45% meaning that 45% of the screened population were in need of a psychiatric examination. If this level of Q is too heavy a burden for the psychiatric service, a higher cut-point can be chosen and the plots will indicate which test is best at this level. The number of false positive individuals is also of concern in a screening program and the false alarm rate 1-SP appears in the plots.

No screening instrument performed well with regard to the detection of somatoform disorders. This may be due to the fact that a sample of persons on LSA includes persons with physical and mental disorders. This may impose problems to SCL-SOM which rates somatic symptoms only. The frequent specific musculoskeletal, cardiac and pulmonary disorders in LSA intermingle with the same symptoms when they occur as symptoms of mental distress. With regard to Whiteley-7, worries about sickness due to somatic disorders intermingle with worries originating from somatoform disorders.

## What Implications Do the Analyses Entail for a Screening Program?

The Central Jutland LSA study pointed out the eligible group for screening, namely individuals sick-listed without a psychiatric sick-leave diagnosis and from full time work. In addition, the results of the study demonstrated the importance of deciding at what level a positive test falls within the framework of the screening program.

The implementation of a screening program involves the establishment a policy for screening, the establishment of an organisation, leadership of the program, and quality assurance of the program. However, these issues are beyond the scope of the Central Jutland LSA study and will therefore not be discussed in this chapter.

It is the responsibility of a program to secure that as many individuals as possible from the eligible group participate in the program. The Central Jutland LSA Study had a low participation rate of 46.4% indicating opposition to participate. In general, there is a growing opposition from the population in participating in epidemiological studies [111]. When it comes to mental disorders, there is reason to believe that fear of stigmatisation is a significant issue. The response from more potential participants in the Central Jutland LSA study refusing to participate said that the study not was of relevance for them and that they feared being stigmatized with a mental disorder. This was supported by the study applying multiple imputation for missing values which showed that the frequency of mental disorders was quite as high among nonparticipants as among participants [33]. This implies that a screening program should include public information concerning stigmatisation and the intent with screening. This also indicates that the officers responsible for screening must be educated about these topics as also mentioned earlier.

## Bias

The evaluation of the efficiency of a screening program is affected by three kinds of bias [39]:

- The "Healthy Screenee Effect"
- Lead-Time bias
- Length-Time bias

### *The "Healthy Screenee Effect"*

The healthy screenee effect is a selection bias which jeopardizes the generalisability of screening studies. The selection bias refers to the situation in which the healthiest, best educated, affluent, and physically fit individuals are most likely to be screened which is considered a bias as these individuals are also expected to present with the best outcome. Consequently, the effectiveness of screening would be overestimated. This is considered to be the primary bias of the Central Jutland LSA Study since the randomisation of individuals took place after the participants were screened. It is, furthermore, likely that the individuals who were less affected by psychological distress or individuals that felt the study irrelevant to them were the ones who declined participation in the study. This bias will jeopardize the generalisability of the study to the whole population of sick-listed individuals. If it was the healthiest individuals who participated, the study underestimates the prevalence of mental disorders, and it overestimates the effect on health outcome parameters and economic efficiency. In contrast, if it was the least healthy who participated, the bias is naturally opposite. The non-participation rate was 53.6% so the bias may be considerable. To compensate for this multiple imputation was carried out on the missing cases by means of data from public registers. The results indicated that the prevalence of CMD was slightly higher among non-participants than among participants [33]. This indicates that the study was biased by *the "Healthy Screenee Effect"*.

### *Lead-Time Bias*

Lead time is the interval between the diagnosis of a disease at screening and the time at which the disease would have been detected via the onset of clinical symptoms. If the outcome parameter is the length of time from the time of diagnosis until return to work, lead time bias will occur due to the fact that the screened individuals are diagnosed earlier compared to individuals who are diagnosed at the time of manifest clinical symptoms. The bias will overestimate the efficiency. The bias will be controlled in RCT studies randomising to a screening group and a control group and again when counting time from the time of randomisation for all individuals in the intervention group and the control group. The Central Jutland LSA study did not randomize before the randomisation, but after with regard to the psychiatric examination. However, the intervention group and the control group are, in any other respect than the intervention, identical. Time was noted from the point of randomisation. Consequently, the study is not affected by lead time bias.

***Length-Time Bias***

Length-time bias refers to the overrepresentation among screening-detected cases of those diseases with long preclinical phases as it is supposed that those with a long preclinical phase have a better prognosis. With reference to the Central Jutland LSA study, this bias will not occur in the comparison of the intervention group and control group. However, the generalisability to all individuals on LSA may be biased as the individuals with a slower developing disease may be overrepresented in the study.

## Strengths and Limitations of the Study

It is a strength of the study that all sick-listed individuals on LSA could be identified based on public registers via the Danish social security scheme of paying sickness benefits. However, this identification might not be so easy in countries where sickness absence benefits are based on private insurance or insurance paid by employers.

It is a limitation of the study that the response rate was only 46.4%. The non-participation rate of the study, however, is frequently met in studies of sickness absence as evident in other studies showing rates of similar magnitude or even higher [112-116]. The study compensated for non-participation by applying multiple imputation for missing values.

The delay concerning the completion of the psychiatric examinations may have induced a bias since a mental disorder could have developed after the sick-listing. This will overestimate the prevalence of undetected mental disorders in relation to the beginning of the sickness absence period. However, at the point in time when entering LSA the prevalence will be representative, and it is usually at this time the rehabilitation programs are commenced.

The coding of sick-leave diagnoses according to the ICPC-classification was carried out by the investigator. Some information specifying a diagnosis may have been lost. However, it is not probable that the differentiation between mental and somatic sick-leave diagnoses was a problem.

The RCT did not examine if and to which degree the recommendations to the general practitioners and rehabilitation services were followed. If the recommendations were not followed, it is possible that the rate of return to work was underestimated. This could be an issue for detailed study based on Danish public registers [107-110].

# Conclusion

CMDs are suitable for screening. The symptom scale SCL-8AD, composed of SCL-ANX4, SCL-8, and SCL-DEP6, was a good screening instrument in screening for anxiety and especially for depression. No instruments were found suitably well in screening for somatoform disorder, not even the specific symptom scales SCL-SOM and Whiteley-7. Plots of SE and 1-SP against Q are more helpful than summary statistics from ROC analyses and QROC analyses when deciding what screening instrument to employ on the basis of best performance at a given level of a positive test. This is quite relevant because the level of a positive test indicates what proportion of the screened population that needs to be followed up with a psychiatric examination, and, subsequently, this group of people must be attended to by psychiatric services, where resources are often limited.

# References

[1] Wittchen HU, Jacobi F. Size and burden of mental disorders in Europe - a critical review and appraisal of 27 studies. *Eur Neuropsychopharmacol* 2005 Aug;15(4):357-76.

[2] Soegaard HJ, Bech P. Psychiatric disorders in long-term sickness absence - a population based cross-sectional study. *Scand J Public Health* 2009;37(7):682-9.

[3] Bijl RV, Ravelli A. Current and residual functional disability associated with psychopathology: findings from the Netherlands Mental Health Survey and Incidence Study (NEMESIS). *Psychol Med* 2000 May;30(3):657-68.

[4] Hays RD, Wells KB, Sherbourne CD, Rogers W, Spritzer K. Functioning and well-being outcomes of patients with depression compared with chronic general medical illnesses. *Arch Gen Psychiatry* 1995 Jan;52(1):11-9.

[5] Sherbourne CD, Wells KB, Judd LL. Functioning and well-being of patients with panic disorder. *Am J Psychiatry* 1996 Feb;153(2):213-8.

[6] Sobieraj M, Williams J, Marley J, Ryan P. The impact of depression on the physical health of family members. *Br J Gen Pract* 1998 Oct;48 (435):1653-5.

[7] Wells KB, Stewart A, Hays RD, Burnam MA, Rogers W, Daniels M, et al. The functioning and well-being of depressed patients. Results from the Medical Outcomes Study. *JAMA* 1989 Aug 18;262(7):914-9.

[8] Bass C, Peveler R, House A. Somatoform disorders: severe psychiatric illnesses neglected by psychiatrists. *Br J Psychiatry* 2001 Jul;179:11-4.

[9] Cassano P, Fava M. Depression and public health: an overview. *J Psychosom Res* 2002 Oct;53(4):849-57.

[10] Andlin-Sobocki P, Jonsson B, Wittchen HU, Olesen J. Cost of disorders of the brain in Europe. *Eur J Neurol* 2005 Jun;12 Suppl 1:1-27.

[11] Hiller W, Rief W, Fichter MM. How disabled are patients with somatoform disorders? *Gen Hosp Psychiatry* 1997 Nov;19(6):432-8.

[12] Murray CJ, Lopez AD. Global mortality, disability, and the contribution of risk factors: Global Burden of Disease Study. *Lancet* 1997 May 17;349(9063):1436-42.

[13] Ladwig KH, Marten-Mittag B, Erazo N, Gundel H. Identifying somatization disorder in a population-based health examination survey: psychosocial burden and gender differences. *Psychosomatics* 2001 Nov;42(6):511-8.

[14] Creed F, Barsky A. A systematic review of the epidemiology of somatisation disorder and hypochondriasis. *J Psychosom Res* 2004 Apr;56(4):391-408.

[15] Lepine JP, Gastpar M, Mendlewicz J, Tylee A. Depression in the community: the first pan-European study DEPRES (Depression Research in European Society). *Int Clin Psychopharmacol* 1997 Jan;12(1):19-29.

[16] OECD. Sickness, Disability and Work: Keeping on track in the economic downturn - background paper. 2009. http:r//www.oecd.org/dataoecd/42/15/42699911.pdf.

[17] Hensing G, Andersson L, Brage S. Increase in sickness absence with psychiatric diagnosis in Norway: a general population-based epidemiologic study of age, gender and regional distribution. *BMC Med* 2006;4:19.

[18] Paykel ES, Priest RG. Recognition and management of depression in general practice: consensus statement. *BMJ* 1992 Nov 14;305(6863):1198-202.

[19] Christensen KS, Toft T, Frostholm L, Ornbol E, Fink P, Olesen F. Screening for common mental disorders: who will benefit? Results from a randomised clinical trial. *Fam Pract* 2005 Aug;22(4):428-34.

[20] Munk-Jorgensen P, Fink P, Brevik JI, Dalgard OS, Engberg M, Hansson L, et al. Psychiatric morbidity in primary public health care: a multicentre investigation. Part II. Hidden morbidity and choice of treatment. *Acta Psychiatr Scand* 1997 Jan;95(1):6-12.

[21] Overland S, Glozier N, Krokstad S, Mykletun A. Undertreatment before the award of a disability pension for mental illness: the HUNT Study. *Psychiatr Serv* 2007 Nov;58(11):1479-82.

[22] Mykletun A, Overland S, Dahl AA, Krokstad S, Bjerkeset O, Glozier N, et al. A population-based cohort study of the effect of common mental disorders on disability pension awards. *Am J Psychiatry* 2006 Aug;163(8):1412-8.

[23] Honkonen TI, Aro TA, Isometsa ET, Virtanen EM, Katila HO. Quality of treatment and disability compensation in depression: comparison of 2 nationally representative samples with a 10-year interval in Finland. *J Clin Psychiatry* 2007 Dec;68(12):1886-93.

[24] Gilbody S, House AO, Sheldon TA. Screening and case finding instruments for depression. *Cochrane Database Syst Rev* 2005;(4): CD002792.

[25] Gilbody SM, House AO, Sheldon TA. Routinely administered questionnaires for depression and anxiety: systematic review. *BMJ* 2001 Feb 17;322(7283):406-9.

[26] Olaya-Contreras P, Persson T, Styf P. Comparison between the Beck Depression Inventory and psychiatric evaluation of distress in patients on long-term sickness leave due to chronic musculoskeletal pain. *Journal of Multidisciplinary Healthcare* 2010;3:161-7.

[27] Hensing G, Spak F. Psychiatric disorders as a factor in sick-leave due to other diagnoses. A general population-based study. *Br J Psychiatry* 1998 Mar;172:250-6.

[28] Stansfeld S, Feeney A, Head J, Canner R, North F, Marmot M. Sickness absence for psychiatric illness: the Whitehall II Study. *Soc Sci Med* 1995 Jan;40(2):189-97.

[29] Hickie IB, Davenport TA, Ricci CS. Screening for depression in general practice and related medical settings. *Med J Aust* 2002 Oct 7;177 Suppl:S111-S116.

[30] Pignone MP, Gaynes BN, Rushton JL, Burchell CM, Orleans CT, Mulrow CD, et al. Screening for depression in adults: a summary of the evidence for the U.S. Preventive Services Task Force. *Ann Intern Med* 2002 May 21;136(10):765-76.

(31) Soegaard H.J. Undetected Common Mental Disorders in Long-Term Sickness Absence. International J Fam Medicine 2012. doi:10.1155 /2012/474989

[32] Soegaard HJ. Choosing screening instrument and cut-point on screening instruments. A comparison of methods. *Scand J Public Health* 2009;37(8):872-80.

[33] Soegaard HJ, Pedersen P. Prevalence of common mental disorders among incident individuals on long-term sickness absence when compensating for non-participation. *Psychology* 2012 in press.

[34] Soegaard HJ, Bech P. Psychometric Analysis of Common Mental Disorders - Screening Questionnaire (CMD-SQ]in Long-Term Sickness Absence. *Scand J Public Health* 2009;37(8):855-63.

[35] Soegaard HJ, Bech P. The effect on length of sickness absence by recognition of undetected psychiatric disorder in long-term sickness absence. A randomized controlled trial. *Scand J Public Health* 2009;37(8):864-71.

[36] Soegaard HJ, Bech P. Compensating for non-response in a study estimating the incidence of mental disorders in long-term sickness absence by a two-phased design. *Scand J Pub Health* 2009;38(6):625-32.

[37] Soegaard HJ, Bech P. Predictive validity of Common Mental Disorders Screening Questionnaire as screening Instrument in Long-term Sickness Absence. *Scand J Public Health* 2010;38(4):375-85.

[38] Soegaard HJ, Bech P. The effect of detecting undetected common mental disorders on psychological distress and quality of life in long-term sickness absence. A randomized controlled trial. *Scand J Public Health* 2010;38(8):845-56.

[39] Raffle A, Gray M. Screening. Evidence and Practice. New York: Oxford University Press; 2007.

[40] Wilson JMG, Jungner G. Principles and Pratice of Screening for disease. Geneva: World Health Organization; 1968.

[41] Eddy DM. How to think about screening. In: Eddy DM, editor. Common screening tests. 1st ed. Philadelphia: *American College of Physicians*; 1991. p. 1-21.

[42] Herman CR, Harmindar KG, Eng J, Fajardo LL. Screening for Preclinical Disease: Test and Disease Characteristics. Fundamentals of Clinical Research for Radiologists 2002;825-31.

[43] Christensen KS, Toft T, Frostholm L, Ornbol E, Fink P, Olesen F. The FIP study: a randomised, controlled trial of screening and recognition of psychiatric disorders. *Br J Gen Pract* 2003 Oct;53(495):758-63.

[44] Christensen KS. Screening for functional and mental disorders in general practice. Results from a randomised clinical trial Research Unit for Functional Disorders, Aarhus University Hospital and Research Unit and Department of General Practice, Faculty of Health Sciences, University of Aarhus; 2004.

[45] Christensen KS, Fink P, Toft T, Frostholm L, Ornbol E, Olesen F. A brief case-finding questionnaire for common mental disorders: the CMDQ. *Fam Pract* 2005 Aug;22(4):448-57.

[46] Goldberg D, Bridges K. Screening for psychiatric illness in general practice: the general practitioner versus the screening questionnaire. *J R Coll Gen Pract* 1987 Jan;37(294):15-8.

[47] Goldberg DP, Gater R, Sartorius N, Ustun TB, Piccinelli M, Gureje O, et al. The validity of two versions of the GHQ in the WHO study of mental illness in general health care. *Psychol Med* 1997 Jan;27(1):191-7.

[48] Spitzer RL, Williams JB, Kroenke K, Linzer M, deGruy FV, III, Hahn SR, et al. Utility of a new procedure for diagnosing mental disorders in primary care. The PRIME-MD 1000 study. *JAMA* 1994 Dec 14;272(22):1749-56.

[49] Spitzer RL, Kroenke K, Williams JB. Validation and utility of a self-report version of PRIME-MD: the PHQ primary care study. Primary Care Evaluation of Mental Disorders. Patient Health Questionnaire. *JAMA* 1999 Nov 10;282(18):1737-44.

[50] Weissman MM, Broadhead WE, Olfson M, Sheehan DV, Hoven C, Conolly P, et al. A diagnostic aid for detecting (DSM-IV]mental disorders in primary care. *Gen Hosp Psychiatry* 1998 Jan;20(1):1-11.

[51] Derogatis LR. SCL-90-R. Administration, Scoring, and Procedures. MANUAL-II. Towson, MD: Clinical Psychometric Research; 1983.

[52] Fink P, Ornbol E, Hansen MS, Sondergaard L, De Jonge P. Detecting mental disorders in general hospitals by the SCL-8 scale. *J Psychosom Res* 2004 Mar;56(3):371-5.

[53] Fink P, Ewald H, Jensen J, Sorensen L, Engberg M, Holm M, et al. Screening for somatization and hypochondriasis in primary care and neurological in-patients: a seven-item scale for hypochondriasis and somatization. *J Psychosom Res* 1999 Mar;46(3):261-73.

[54] Fiellin DA, Reid MC, O'Connor PG. Screening for alcohol problems in primary care: a systematic review. *Arch Intern Med* 2000 Jul 10;160(13):1977-89.

[55] Holi M. Assessment of psychiatric symptoms using SCL-90 Department of Psychiatry, Helsinki University, Finland; 2003.

[56] The International Classification of Primary Care in the European Community. Oxford: Oxford University Press; 1993.

[57] Bass C, Peveler R, House A. Somatoform disorders: severe psychiatric illnesses neglected by psychiatrists. *Br J Psychiatry* 2001 Jul;179:11-4.

[58] Weissman MM, Wickramaratne P, Nomura Y, Warner V, Pilowsky D, Verdeli H. Offspring of depressed parents: 20 years later. *Am J Psychiatry* 2006 Jun;163(6):1001-8.

[59] Garber J. Depression in children and adolescents: linking risk research and prevention. *Am J Prev Med* 2006 Dec;31(6 Suppl 1):S104-S125.

[60] Bostwick JM, Pankratz VS. Affective disorders and suicide risk: a reexamination. *Am J Psychiatry* 2000 Dec;157(12):1925-32.

[61] Hoyer EH, Mortensen PB, Olesen AV. Mortality and causes of death in a total national sample of patients with affective disorders admitted for the first time between 1973 and 1993. *Br J Psychiatry* 2000 Jan;176:76-82.

[62] Kessler RC, Ormel J, Demler O, Stang PE. Comorbid mental disorders account for the role impairment of commonly occurring chronic physical disorders: results from the National Comorbidity Survey. *J Occup Environ Med* 2003 Dec;45(12):1257-66.

[63] Kessing LV, Forman JL, Andersen PK. Do continued antidepressants protect against dementia in patients with severe depressive disorder? *Int Clin Psychopharmacol* 2011 Nov;26(6):316-22.

[64] Hasselbalch BJ, Knorr U, Kessing LV. Cognitive impairment in the remitted state of unipolar depressive disorder: a systematic review. *J Affect Disord* 2011 Nov;134(1-3):20-31.

[65] Kessing LV, Forman JL, Andersen PK. Does lithium protect against dementia? *Bipolar Disord* 2010 Feb;12(1):87-94.

[66] Kessing LV, Sondergard L, Forman JL, Andersen PK. Antidepressants and dementia. *J Affect Disord* 2009 Sep;117(1-2):24-9.

[67] Trichard C, Martinot JL, Alagille M, Masure MC, Hardy P, Ginestet D, et al. Time course of prefrontal lobe dysfunction in severely depressed in-patients: a longitudinal neuropsychological study. *Psychol Med* 1995 Jan;25(1):79-85.

[68] Reischies FM, Neu P. Comorbidity of mild cognitive disorder and depression--a neuropsychological analysis. *Eur Arch Psychiatry Clin Neurosci* 2000;250(4):186-93.

[69] Jorm AF. Is depression a risk factor for dementia or cognitive decline? A review. *Gerontology* 2000 Jul;46(4):219-27.

[70] Jorm AF. History of depression as a risk factor for dementia: an updated review. *Aust N Z J Psychiatry* 2001 Dec;35(6):776-81.

[71] Hasselbalch BJ, Knorr U, Hasselbalch SG, Gade A, Kessing LV. Cognitive Deficits in the Remitted State of Unipolar Depressive Disorder. *Neuropsychology* 2012 Jul 23.

[72] World Health Organisation. International Statistical Classification of Diseases and Related Health Problems. 10th Revision. Geneve: World Health Organisation; 2006.

[73] American Psychiatric Association. The *Diagnostic and Statistical Manual of Mental Disorders, Fourth Edition* (*DSM-IV*). American Psychiatric Association 2011. Available from: URL: http://psych.org/MainMenu/Research/DSMIV.aspx

[74] Sartorius N, Ustun TB, Lecrubier Y, Wittchen HU. Depression comorbid with anxiety: results from the WHO study on psychological disorders in primary health care. *Br J Psychiatry Suppl* 1996 Jun;(30): 38-43.

[75] Fava GA. Subclinical symptoms in mood disorders: pathophysiological and therapeutic implications. *Psychol Med* 1999 Jan;29(1):47-61.

[76] Fava GA, Mangelli L. Assessment of subclinical symptoms and psychological well-being in depression. *Eur Arch Psychiatry Clin Neurosci* 2001;251 Suppl 2:II47-II52.

[77] Rutter M, Kim-Cohen J, Maughan B. Continuities and discontinuities in psychopathology between childhood and adult life. *J Child Psychol Psychiatry* 2006 Mar;47(3-4):276-95.

[78] Rydmark I, Wahlberg K, Ghatan PH, Modell S, Nygren A, Ingvar M, et al. Neuroendocrine, cognitive and structural imaging characteristics of women on longterm sickleave with job stress-induced depression. *Biol Psychiatry* 2006 Oct 15;60(8):867-73.

[79] Olsen LR, Mortensen EL, Bech P. Prevalence of major depression and stress indicators in the Danish general population. *Acta Psychiatr Scand* 2004 Feb;109(2):96-103.

[80] Frank E, Judge R. Treatment recommendations versus treatment realities: recognizing the rift and understanding the consequences. *J Clin Psychiatry* 2001;62 Suppl 22:10-5.

[81] Judd LL. The clinical course of unipolar major depressive disorders. *Arch Gen Psychiatry* 1997 Nov;54(11):989-91.

[82] Mueller TI, Leon AC, Keller MB, Solomon DA, Endicott J, Coryell W, et al. Recurrence after recovery from major depressive disorder during 15 years of observational follow-up. *Am J Psychiatry* 1999 Jul;156(7):1000-6.

[83] Kessing LV, Hansen MG, Andersen PK, Angst J. The predictive effect of episodes on the risk of recurrence in depressive and bipolar disorders - a life-long perspective. *Acta Psychiatr Scand* 2004 May;109(5):339-44.

[84] Keller MB, Lavori PW, Mueller TI, Endicott J, Coryell W, Hirschfeld RM, et al. Time to recovery, chronicity, and levels of psychopathology in major depression. A 5-year prospective follow-up of 431 subjects. *Arch Gen Psychiatry* 1992 Oct;49(10):809-16.

[85] Mitte K, Noack P, Steil R, Hautzinger M. A meta-analytic review of the efficacy of drug treatment in generalized anxiety disorder. *J Clin Psychopharmacol* 2005 Apr;25(2):141-50.

[86] Mitte K. A meta-analysis of the efficacy of psycho- and pharma-cotherapy in panic disorder with and without agoraphobia. *J Affect Disord* 2005 Sep;88(1):27-45.

[87] Mitte K. Meta-analysis of cognitive-behavioral treatments for generalized anxiety disorder: a comparison with pharmacotherapy. *Psychol Bull* 2005 Sep;131(5):785-95.

[88] Sondergard L, Lopez AG, Andersen PK, Kessing LV. Mood-stabilizing pharmacological treatment in bipolar disorders and risk of suicide. *Bipolar Disord* 2008 Feb;10(1):87-94.

[89] Sondergard L, Lopez AG, Andersen PK, Kessing LV. Continued antidepressant treatment and suicide in patients with depressive disorder. *Arch Suicide Res* 2007;11(2):163-75.

[90] World Federation of Socities of Biological Psychiatry. S3-Guideline/National Disease Management Guideline. Unipolar Depression. Short version. 2012. Ref Type: Internet Communication

[91] National Institute for Health and Clinical Excellence. Nice Guidance. *Social anxiety disorder*. 2012.

[92] National Institute for Health and Clinical Excellence. Management of anxiety (panic disorders with or without agoraphobia, and generalised anxiety disorder]in adults in primary care, secondary and community care. 2012.

[93] McEwen BS. Allostasis and allostatic load: implications for neuropsychopharmacology. *Neuropsychopharmacology* 2000 Feb;22(2):108-24.

[94] Cronbach LJ, Meehl PE. Construct validity in psychological tests. Psychol Bull 1955 Jul;52(4):281-302.

[95] SCAN. Schedules for Clinical Assessment in Neuropsychiatry [computer program]. Geneva.: World Health Organization; 1994.

[96] Kraemer HC. Evaluating Medical Tests: Objective and Quantitative Guidelines. Newbury Park, CA: SAGE Publications; 1992.

[97] Tape, TG.The Area Under an ROC Curve: http://gim.unmc.edu/dxtests/ROC3.htm. 2007.

[98] Viera AJ, Garrett JM. Understanding interoberver Agreement: The Kappa Sttatistic. *Fam Med* 2012;37(5):360-3.

[99] Mokken R. A Theory and Procedure of Scale Analysis. The Hague. The Netherlands: Mouton; 1971.

[100] Olsen LR, Mortensen EL, Bech P. The SCL-90 and SCL-90R versions validated by item response models in a Danish community sample. *Acta Psychiatr Scand* 2004 Sep;110(3):225-9.

[101] Bjørner JB, Damsgaard MT, Watt T, Bech P, Rasmussen NK, Kristensen TS, et al. Dansk Manual til SF-36. Et spørgeskema om helbredsstatus. København: Lægemiddel Industri Foreningen; 1997.

[102] Ware JE, Kosinski M. SF-36 Physical and Mental Health Summary Scales: A Manual for Users of Version 1. 2nd ed. Lincoln,RI: Quality Metric, Inc.; 2001.

[103] Valenstein M, Vijan S, Zeber JE, Boehm K, Buttar A. The cost-utility of screening for depression in primary care. *Ann Intern Med* 2001 Mar 6;134(5):345-60.

[104] Arbejdsmarkedsstyrelsen, The National Labour Market authority. DREAM-databasen. The DREAM Databse. http://www.dst.dk/TilSalg/Forskningsservice/Databaser/Dream.aspx.

[105] Det Centrale Personregister.The Civil Registration System in Denmark. Det Centrale Personregister. The Civil Registration System in Denmark. http://www.cpr.dk/cpr/site.aspx?p=198&ArticleTypeID=76&t=ForsideVisartikel&Articleid=4327.

[106] The National Board of Health D. The National Board of Health, Denmark. http://www.sst.dk/English.aspx.

[107] The National Board of Health D. Lægemiddeldatabasen. The medication database http://www.dst.dk/TilSalg/Forskningsservice/ Databaser/LMDB/LMDBdata.aspx.

[108] Galea S, Tracy M. Participation rates in epidemiologic studies. *Ann Epidemiol* 2007 Sep;17(9):643-53.

[109] Duijts SF, Kant I, van den Brandt PA, Swaen GM. Effectiveness of a preventive coaching intervention for employees at risk for sickness absence due to psychosocial health complaints: results of a randomized controlled trial. *J Occup Environ Med* 2008 Jul;50(7):765-76.

[110] Huibers MJ, Beurskens AJ, Van Schayck CP, Bazelmans E, Metsemakers JF, Knottnerus JA, et al. Efficacy of cognitive-behavioural therapy by general practitioners for unexplained fatigue among employees: Randomised controlled trial. *Br J Psychiatry* 2004 Mar;184:240-6.

[111] Proper KI, van der Beek AJ, Hildebrandt VH, Twisk JW, van Mechelen W. Worksite health promotion using individual counselling and the effectiveness on sick leave; results of a randomised controlled trial. *Occup Environ Med* 2004 Mar;61(3):275-9.

[112] Taimela S, Justen S, Aronen P, Sintonen H, Laara E, Malmivaara A, et al. An occupational health intervention programme for workers at high risk for sickness absence. Cost effectiveness analysis based on a randomised controlled trial. *Occup Environ Med* 2008 Apr;65(4):242-8.

[113] Taimela S, Malmivaara A, Justen S, Laara E, Sintonen H, Tiekso J, et al. The effectiveness of two occupational health intervention programmes in reducing sickness absence among employees at risk. Two randomised controlled trials. *Occup Environ Med* 2008 Apr;65(4):236-41.

In: Screening Tests
Editor: Marguerite Gauthier

ISBN: 978-1-62417-963-1
© 2013 Nova Science Publishers, Inc.

*Chapter 2*

# A VISION SCREENING TEST TO NEWBORNS

***Merce Leonhardt*[1,*], *Maria Forns*[2] *and Caterina Calderón*[2]**

[1]NICU, Hospital Sant Pau, Cartagena, s/n. Barcelona, Spain
[2]Deparment of Personality, Assessment and Psychological Treatment, Faculty of Psychology, University of Barcelona, Spain

## ABSTRACT

The early detection of visual disorders is important in order to minimize the consequences of visual impairment or delayed visual maturation, especially in newborn or preterm children with and without other disorders such as brain injuries or heart disease. The implementation of early intervention programs is essential.

Research has provided evidence that certain visual abilities are present from birth. Instruments designed to detect these abilities include those created by Atkinson's and Ricci's teams and the ML-Leonhardt Optotype Battery which assesses visual functions and distinguishes between reflex and perceptive vision.

This chapter describes the ML-Leonhardt Optotype Battery and discusses the results obtained interm and preterm newborns with and without injuries. The data indicate that preterm infants with brain lesions

* Corresponding author Merçè Leonhardt, NICU, Hospital Sant Joan de Déu. Passeig Sant Joan de Déu, 2. Esplugues 08950. Barcelona, Spain. NICU, Hospital Vall d'Hebron. Passeig Vall d'Hebron, 119-129. 08035 Barcelona, Spain. Email address: sanleon@pangea.org Phone +34935831532; Fax +34934021362.

showed a delayed pattern of visual functions in alertness, fixation, visual attention and tracking behavior when compared to healthy preterm infants of around 30%. These visual functions can be identified in the first weeks of life.

This early period in life is characterized by enormous sensitivity. When a visual disorder is detected, the initiation of visual stimulation enhances the infant's potential for change. A multidisciplinary approach involving neonatologists, ophthalmologists and neurologists is key to early detection.

## 1. INTRODUCTION

Several studies have addressed the assessment of various aspects of visual function in preterm and term-born infants [1, 2, 3] by focusing on the early detection of visual disorders. The visual system is the integrator of the sense perceptual experiences that provide the baby with a mental representation. Good visual system performance from very early stages is necessary to the optimal development of the cognitive functions linked to the visual system. Therefore, neonatologists and psychologists specializing in early infancy should have access to instruments able to assessment visual function in the newborn.

The assessment of visual function in newborn infants explores various aspects, ranging from alertness to the ability to track a stimulus. This assessment is now part of most neurological examinations. An example is the Amiel-Tison standardized neonatal neurological assessment [4], which records information about the type of ocular movements, visual alertness (in response to a red ball or black and white target) and the ability to fix and follow the same target horizontally, vertically, or in a complete arc. The Brazelton neonatal behavioral assessment scale [5] also examines visual alertness, as well as orientation to animate or inanimate visual targets.

The early detection of visual disorders can help to minimize the consequences of visual impairment, especially in children with brain injury [6, 7]. Studies of infants with brain lesions have reported the correlation between specific aspects of visual function and lesions affecting anatomical structures in the visual pathway using magnetic resonance imaging (MRI) [8, 9, 10], visual evoked potentials (VEP) [11] and batteries of optotypes [2, 12].

Many preterm infants are at a higher risk of neurodevelopmental and visual impairment than term-born infants. Visual deficits may be due to retinopathy of prematurity, or to brain lesions in the optic pathways and associated areas [13]. Mercuri et al [7] and Atkinson et al. [12] have provided evidence that early visual abilities are present in both preterm and full-term new-born children, and have described a functioning model of the diverse systems that are involved in vision.

Recently, Ricci et al. [14] described a visual test battery which included nine stimuli that assess ocular movements (spontaneous behavior and behavior in response to a target), the ability to fix and follow a black/white target (horizontally, vertically, and in an arc), the reaction to a colored target, the ability to discriminate black and white stripes of increasing spatial frequency, and the ability to keep attention on a black and white target that is slowly moving away from the infant. Ricci and her research group conducted an in-depth exploration of visual function by applying a newly-developed clinical assessment battery to a cohort of low risk-full-term newborns [2, 15]. Their findings showed that around 90% of low-risk term-born newborn could conjugate ocular motility, showed stable fixation, could track patterns horizontally, vertically and in an arc, reacted to tracking colored stimulus, discriminated between black and white stripes (0.86 cycles/degree or higher) and maintained attention on a distant stimulus. These authors compared preterm visual function at term-equivalent age with those of term-born infants [16]. They found that the early extra uterine experience of low-risk infants of 35 to 40 weeks post-menstrual age accelerated the maturation of visual function as regards stability and tracking. In their longitudinal assessment of visual function in low-risk preterm infants at 3, 5 and 12 months [17], they found that more than 85% of infants were able to fix and follow a target, and presented normal results on acuity, visual fields, and attention at distance. These results suggest that the maturation of these visual functions was not affected by preterm birth when adjusted for prematurity.

Guzzeta et al. [13] and Mercuri et al. [7] assess visual function using electrophysiological techniques. They offer data concerning blink reflex, oculomotor behavior, acuity, visual fields, optokinetic nystagmus, fixation and visual evoked potential shift. They also use neuroimaging to detect visual impairments in children with brain damage, though they report that the lesions do not always correspond to the child's functionality.

The behavioral aspects of visual function have mainly been studied after the neonatal period, when more mature aspects of this function can be assessed [18]. Using the Atkinson Battery of Child Development for Examining Functional Vision (ABCDEFV) with infants from 0 to 4 years old, Atkinson et al. [12] demonstrated the importance of visual function for child development.

Leonhardt [19, 20] reported the use of the *ML-Leonhardt Optotype Battery* to explore visual functions in low-risk preterm newborns. These authors assessed visual responses in 50 term and 130 preterm newborns aged between three and 48 days using optotypes and the human face. It was found that preterm infants reacted to the visual stimulus, performing responses of alertness, fixation and tracking to the human face and to the high- and low-contrast optotypes.

The study concluded that both preterm and term newborns showed visual abilities from birth. Between 80% and 100% of term infants showed alertness and fixation to the stimulus, and between 75% and 95% were able to attend to the stimulus [21]. The study concluded that visual functions are present from a very early stage.

# 2. Measurement of the Visual Function in Neonates

Instruments that systematically measure the visual function in neonates are scarce. Here, we highlight two relevant recent instruments specifically designed to assess visual functions: Ricci's battery [15], and Atkinson's ABCDEFV battery[12]. We also refer briefly to Brazelton's scale [22].

## 2.1. Ricci et al.'s Battery

Ricci and colleagues [15] developed a clinical instrument for assessing visual function in newborn infants which can be applied to children from the age of 48 hours.

This instrument analyses: a) spontaneous visual behavior, b) visual behavior elicited by the presence of various optotypes, c) fixation, d) tracking behavior of optotype movements (in horizontal, vertical and in an arc), e) the tracking reaction to color, f) the discrimination of optotypes of different widths, and g) attention to distance. The test should be applied in behavioral state 4 or 5 in the classification proposed by Brazelton [23].

The protocol comprises the following visual functions:

a) *Spontaneous visual behavior*: two aspects are analyzed:

a.1. *Spontaneous ocular motility* which considers the following eye movements: conjugation, strabismus and nystagmus, measured as occasional, intermittent or predominant. Ninety per cent of infants have conjugated ocular motility with occasional nystagmus or strabismus (2.5%) at 48 hours.

a.2. *Fixation.* Ninety-two per cent of neonates show fixation and 7.8% present isolation at 48 hours.

b) *Visual behavior elicited by the presence of cards:* an optotype with black and white concentric circular lines is used to elicit visual behavior.
The diameter of the optotype is 10 cm, and each stripe is 1.8 cm. wide (in accordance with the Amiel-Tison model). Ocular motility, fixing and tracking are analyzed. The card is presented at a distance of 20-30 cm from the child's face.

b.1. *Motility:* Sixty per cent of children conjugate eye movements and 34.5% show occasional strabismus or nystagmus.

b.2. *Fixation:* stable (> 3 seconds) in 99% of children, and unstable (< 3 seconds) in 1%.

b.3 *Tracking:* the optotype is presented in the central point of the child's visual field and is moved slowly at a speed of $3^{o}$ s. The following behaviors are analyzed:

a) Horizontal tracking (moving to the right and left). Complete in 90% of newborns, incomplete in 7.8%, and brief in 2.2%.
b) Vertical tracking (upward and downward movement). Complete in 67.8% of newborns, incomplete in 28.9%, and brief in 3.3%
c) Arc tracking (arc movement). Complete in 67.8% of newborns, incomplete in 28.8%, and brief in 3.4%

c) The *quality of follow-up* (pursuit behavior) is evaluated as continuous and discontinuous.
d) The *reaction to a colored stimulus* is analyzed through the presentation of a card displaying a yellow and red face. The card measures 15 x 15 cm and the face is 10 cm in diameter. The card is presented at a distance of 25 cm from the newborn. The saccadic movements to center the image on the fovea are assessed, as is the

presence or absence of fixation and tracking of the target. Tracking is observed in 98.8% of newborns.

e) The *discrimination of stripes of different widths* is analyzed through a set of cards obtained from the optotypes proposed by Teller for analyzing visual acuity. Eight cards bearing stripes of decreasing width (ranging from 1.5 to 0.11 cm) are used. Cards are presented at a distance of 38 cm. Ninety-five per cent of infants discriminate stripes with a spatial frequency of 0.86 cycles/degree or higher.

f) *Attention to distance* is evaluated with two optotypes. The first shows a face in black and white, and the second shows a face with high-contrast yellow and red. The target is moved at a slight angle on the horizontal arc in order to avoid possible hyperfixation. More than 95% of infants maintain attention at a distance of 30 cm, with both stimuli.

Reliability of the battery: concordance is above 90% between observers and the senior examiner, and also between individual observers. As a whole this battery is easy to use, requires no specific training, and can be used in the nursery or the intensive care unit, even in incubators. The material required is small and is washable.

The test can be performed in 5/10 minutes. It provides useful information on various aspects of visual function of newborns.

This battery has been used to assess visual function in a population of low risk full term newborns [15], in low risk preterm infants at postmenstrual age of 35 and 40 weeks [15], and in preterm infants with and without brain injury, focusing specifically on visual and neurodevelopmental outcome at 12 months [24].

## 2.2. Battery ABCDEFV by Atkinson et al.'s Battery

The Atkinson battery [12] is a battery that taps to assess early development visual and psychical and social children competencies. This battery have been normalized and standardized for children between birth and four mental age ranges. It analyses visual function by 22 tests: sensory visual measure such as acuity, visual fields and stereopsis, as well as perceptual, motor, spatial and cognitive aspects of visual function. The battery is divided into three parts.

First part analyses the ‘core vision test’ or basic visual capacities in children of any age being able to move head and eye. The visual functions assessed in this core vision test are the following ones: '

- Responsiveness of pupil to the light
- Diffuse light reaction: the orientation to light
- Lateral tracking: the visual attention and eye pursuit
- Peripheral refixation-lateral fields
- Symmetrical corneal reflexes: the binocular alignment
- Converge to approaching object: binocular function
- Attention at distance
- Defensive blink to approaching object
- Visually follows falling toy: visual cognition as development of object permanence

Second part analyses some “optional core vision tests” as reflex eye movements associated with both subcortical and cortical mechanisms, measurement of visual acuity, and accommodation, attention shifts and refractive errors. The optional core vision tests are:

- Optokinetic nystagmus (OKN)
- Acuity cards for preferential looking (Teller/Keller)
- Accomodation (videorefraction)

The third part comprise “additional test” and it is composed by some of the following test

- Lang test of binocular vision (Stereoscopic)
- Batting and reaching: visuo-motor competence
- Pick up black and white cotton threat: visual control of fine hand and finger movement (pincer grasp)
- Visual cognition: intermediate stage in development of object permanence (retrieval of a partially covered or totally covered objet)
- Shape recognition, recognition of spatial relations, visual planning and control of manual actions
- Embedded figures: visuo-cognitive task of perceptual organization. Figure-ground segmentation and shape recognition

**Table 1. Test of Battery ABCDEFV**

| Recommended test[a] | 0-6 weeks | 7-12 weeks | 13-19 weeks | 20-29 weeks | 30-52 weeks | 13-18 months | 19-24 months | 25-30 months | 31-36 months |
|---|---|---|---|---|---|---|---|---|---|
| Pupil responses | 100% | 100% | 100% | 100% | 100% | 100% | 100% | 100% | 100% |
| Diffuse light reaction | 90% | 100% | 100% | | | | | | |
| Symmetrical corneal reflex | 80% | 90% | 100% | 100% | 100% | 100% | 100% | 100% | 100% |
| Convergence | 80% | 90% | 100% | 100% | 100% | 100% | 98% | 100% | 100% |
| Lateral fields | | 90% | 90% | 95% | 100% | | | | |
| Tracking | 90% | 90% | 100% | 100% | 100% | 100% | 100% | 100% | 100% |
| Attention at distance | | | | 90% | 100% | 100% | 100% | 100% | 100% |
| Defensive blink | | 40% | 70% | 100% | 100% | 100% | | | |
| Follow falling toy | | | | 95% | 100% | | | | |
| OKN | | | 90% | 95% | 85% | | | | |
| Acuity cards | 90% | 95% | 90% | 95% | 100% | 100% | 100% | 100% | 100% |
| Video Refraction | 50% | 70% | 70% | 95% | 100% | 100% | 100% | 95% | 95% |
| Lang stereo test | | | | | | | | 80% | 100% |

| Recommended test[a] | 0-6 weeks | 7-12 weeks | 13-19 weeks | 20-29 weeks | 30-52 weeks | 13-18 months | 19-24 months | 25-30 months | 31-36 months |
|---|---|---|---|---|---|---|---|---|---|
| Batting and reaching | | | | 80% | 100% | 100% | 95% | 100% | 100% |
| Pincer grasp of Black/white cotton | | | | | 50% | 100% | 95% | 100% | 100% |
| Partially covered object | | | | 35% | 90% | | | | |
| Totally covered object | | | | 10% | 50% | 80% | | | |
| Shape matching | | | | | | 3 shape 55% | 3 shape test 95% | 5 shape test 85% | 5 shape test 100% |
| Embedded cats and animals | | | | | | 10% | 45% | 95% | 100% |
| Put the card in the envelope | | | | | | | | 30% | 100% |
| Free play blocks | | | | | | 55% | 90% | 80% | 100% |
| Copying block designs | | | | | | * | * | * | * |

[a]Test for each age level marked gray and the different percentages of success according the type of construction (bridge, 77line, etc).

- Placing the letter in the envelope. Recognition of spatial relations, visual planning, and control of manual actions
- Spatial block-construction, in free play situation
- Copying block designs: constructional apraxia.

Some subtest measure spatial vision related to more ventral or more dorsal stream processing, whereas some involve integration across both processing streams.

Normative data are reported for nine age groups between 0-6 weeks and 31-36 months, each including 32-43 typically developing children. The basic battery for each age group can be completed in between 15 and 39 minutes, see table 1.

The ABCDEFV has been applied to a range of at-risk and clinical groups [12]. In large-scale population infant vision screening program (n = 5.000) for detection of strabismus and refractive errors in 9-month-old infants and prevention of later strabismus and amblyopia through spectacle correction in infancy.

## 2.3. Neonatal Behavioural Assessment Scale

The Neonatal Behavioral Assessment Scale [22] is an interactive evaluation technique for assessing newborn behavioral competencies, and to help parents and professionals to understand the newborn's language. When applying the battery parents are taught to understand the contribution of the neonate to the parent-infant system and to accept that the newborn is both competent and organized. It is considered one of the best neonatal scales both for the detection of behavioral and developmental deficits and for the identification of the newborn's emerging capabilities

The *objective of the test* is to offer a picture of the baby's strength, adaptive responses, and competences. This test is also able to identify possible vulnerabilities. In terms of its *structure,* the Brazelton scale comprises two types of items: *35 behavioral and 18 reflex*. Behavioral items are grouped around six factors [22]: 1) autonomic nervous system, 2) motor system, 3) habituation, 4) state organization, 5) state regulation, and 6) social-interactive.

- *Autonomic nervous system.* Integrates the basic functions of the organism such as regulation of breathing and temperature. It comprises three items that analyse tremulousness, startles and lability of the color of the skin.

- *Motor system.* Integrates the motor reactions. It comprises five items. It evaluates the quality of the movements and muscle tone.
- *State regulation.* Analyses newborns' capacity to modulate their states of consciousness. Mechanisms involved are habituation (protection to stimuli that disrupt sleep), consolability (the capacity to be comforted by their parents) and self-quieting.
- *Social-interactive.* When infants achieve a balance in the above systems, they are ready to maintain social interaction, paying attention to stimuli from their environment. This module comprises seven items that assess the capability of the newborn to console himself, and to fix and follow visual and auditory stimuli.

  In the *social-interactive system* there are four specific items that reflect the visual modality of the newborn: 1) inanimate visual orientation (red ball), 2) visual and auditory orientation (rattle), 3) animate visual orientation (examiner's face) and 4) visual and auditory orientation (examiner's face and voice).

All behavioral items are scored on a 9-point Likert scale, with 0 the minimum and 8 the maximum. However, eight items are scored on a curvilinear scale, where the central scores are optimal. These items are coded according to a linear scale of 5, 6 or 8 points. The scores are specific to each item. Reflex responses are measured on a 4-point Likert scale, producing a *profile* that describes the infant's neurobehavioral organization.

*The test is* designed for term neonates from the first hours of life up to 60 days. It can also be applied to preterm infants of less than 37 weeks of gestation; depending on their degree of immaturity, the test may be conducted up to 48 weeks of post gestational age. Items are *administered* in a standard order, though changes are possible. Behavioral and reflex items alternate. During administration, both environmental and physiological conditions must be as favorable as possible to the neonate. *Test duration* is approximately 25 minutes.

### *Application Procedure and Evaluation of Visual Function-Centered Items*

To apply the Brazelton scale the newborn must be in a state of consciousness 4 or 5. The material used comprises a rattle (a red box measuring 10 cm. by 5 cm with small pellets in its interior), a red ball 5 cm. in diameter, and the examiner's face and voice.

a) *Inanimate visual orientation* (red ball) is placed at a distance of 25-30 cm in the middle line, moving slowly and gently to the right and to the left. The examiner must ensure that it does not stay in the field of direct vision of the child but traces a slight arc with regard to the stimulus.
b) *Inanimate visual and auditory orientation* is analyzed using a rattle, which can be used as both a visual and an auditory stimulus. The examiner holds a rattle in front of the child, at an angle of 45 degrees, and at a distance of 25-30 cm approx. The rattle is gently shaken laterally to the child's visual field and is slowly moved into it.
c) *Animate visual orientation* is explored using the examiner's face. The examiner may be either standing or seated but it is important that the newborn's head and body should receive maximum support. Holding the child in the frontal position, at an angle of 45 degrees and a distance of 25-30 cm, the examiner moves the object slowly in a horizontal arc in front of the child. The baby must follow the movement of the examiner's face.
d) *Animate visual auditory orientation* (the examiner's face and voice) is analyzed using the technique described for the animate visual item with the addition of the examiner's voice.

*Evaluation:* The quality of both alert and attention behavior is assessed. The variables are analyzed on a 9-point Likert scale, from 1 (no reaction) and 8 (long-lasting state of alert).

Brazelton's scale [23] is used to identify competences in both healthy and risk infants. Its interactive nature strengthens the link between babies and their parents and enhances infant development [25].

## 3. ML LEONHARDT OPTOTYPE BATTERY FOR NEWBORNS AND AT RISK-INFANTS

The ML Leonhardt Optotype Battery is a screening test for visual functions that analyzes babies' visual response to the presentation of several visual stimuli.

The battery was designed by Leonhardt [21]. It is based on a range of tests of babies' visual sensitivity [12, 22], and specifically on the Brazelton battery; in fact the Leonhardt battery partially reproduces the Brazelton battery's exquisite evaluation system.

The current belief that the visual system of the newborn is mainly subcortical and that in the first months of life it is progressively taken over by cortical processes is supported by the results of specific tests of the visual function in these early ages [26]. The assessment of visual function is part of the standard examination of the newborn, but it is often limited to an ocular examination and to the analysis of basic responses of fixation and tracking of a model of high- contrast concentric circles.

## Objective

The *Leonhardt Optotype Battery* is designed to assess the visual function of term and preterm infants [19, 27, 28] during the first hours of life and to detect any visual disturbances. It may also be administered to older children, especially children with visual deficits and other associated disabilities.

## Material

The test involves fifteen types of visual stimuli. The first stimulus is the human face, followed by seven high-contrast and five low-contrast optotypes. The optotypes are presented on a square base of 11.5 cm.

The first stimulus (human face) serves to analyze the baby's response to the examiner's face. Seven high-contrast optotypes are applied consecutively after the human face. First there are two concentric stimuli. The first optotype comprises three black concentric circles of 1 cm in width [equivalent to 0.50 cycles per degree, as suggested by Teller et al.] [29] against a white background, corresponding to a classical model used in neonatology to assess newborns' visual response. The second optotype is the same, but has squares in place of circles. With these optotypes we observe whether the baby is able to detect the difference in the angles of the figure.

The third and fourth optotypes are black and white horizontal and vertical stripes 2 cm wide (equivalent to 0.25 cycles per degree). This presentation is based on Teller's preferential looking procedure (Teller et al. [29]). In recent decades, these optotypes have been used to measure visual acuity in newborns and preterms.

The fifth and sixth optotypes were narrow black and white horizontal and vertical stripes 1 cm wide (equivalent to 0.50 cycles per degree). The seventh optotype is a drawing of a face in black and white. This design is based on Hÿvarinen et al.'s Visual Test for infants [30] and assesses whether the baby is attracted by the drawing.

All these stimuli are high-contrast. They are followed by five low-contrast optotypes. According to the Bailey-Lovie contrast chart, low-contrast visual acuity (LCVA) is 20% [31]. The eighth optotype is a low-contrast drawing of a face in black and white, which analyses visual acuity sensitivity (as suggested by Hÿvarinen et al. [30].

The ninth and tenth optotypes are low-contrast 2 cm wide black and white horizontal and vertical stripes (equivalent to 0.25 cycles per degree). The eleventh and twelfth optotypes ae narrow, low-contrast black and white horizontal and vertical stripes 1 cm in width (equivalent to 0.50 cycles per degree). The low-contrast optotypes provide information on subjects' contrast sensitivity function.

## Visual Behavioral Responses

The ML Leonhardt Optotype Battery analyzes the visual behavioral responses of alertness, fixation, attention and tracking. Alertness is defined as a minimum visual response to the stimulus presentation. Responses may be very subtle such as a slight inclination toward the stimulus, eye opening, small changes in normal breathing, color changes, and so on, indicating that the baby is aware of the presence of an object.

Fixation is the adaptation of the eyes to converge on the ray of light and obtain a clear image. It is the ability to orient toward a viewed object. Fixation marks the beginning of the attention stage.

The main indicator of fixation behavior is the orientation of vision toward the object. The baby can either look at the stimulus with one eye (monocularly), or with both eyes (binocularly). If during fixation the child changes the focus of one eye but maintains that of the other, this is considered monocular vision.

Attention is defined as maintaining the fixation on the stimulus for at least three seconds. Hyperfixation is not considered as an attention behavior to the object. Alertness, fixation and attention behaviors are coded as 0=absent and 1=present.

Tracking is achieved if the child turns his/her eyes (or eye), or both the head and eyes towards a moving stimulus. Tracking behavior is coded as: A=absent, B=brief (tracking characterized by discontinuous glances), C=incomplete (continuous tracking of the object with the eyes, at an angle of between 30 and 90 degrees), and D=complete (continuous tracking of the object with eyes and head, within the defined angle).

## Conditions of Application

*Adaptation to the baby:* The examiner must adapt to the conditions of fragility and vulnerability of the newborns. Specifically, the battery should be applied gently and slowly, taking care at all times to avoid causing stress to the baby.

The infants are examined while awake and in a calm state (state 4 in Brazelton's classification [22]).

**Table 2. Baby behavior**

| Comfort behavior | Behavior stress |
|---|---|
| Good color skin | Skin color: pale, cyanotic, crosslinked |
| Well maintained, modulated muscle tone | Sagging arms and legs |
| Smooth movements of arms and legs | Motor behavior (extension of arms and legs) |
| Regularity of breath between 40 to 60 bpm | Irregularity of breathing: breathing pauses, slow and/or fast |
| Face relaxed, attempts to move the hand to the mouth, grasping or holding the cloth | Visceral signs (vomiting, choking, hiccups, gasps) |
| Body relaxation | SNA responses (tremor, shocks, spasm) |
| Heart rate between 120 to 160 bpm | Heart rate (less than 120 or more than 160 bpm) |
| Oxygenation saturation between 94 to 98% | Oxygenation saturation less than 90% |

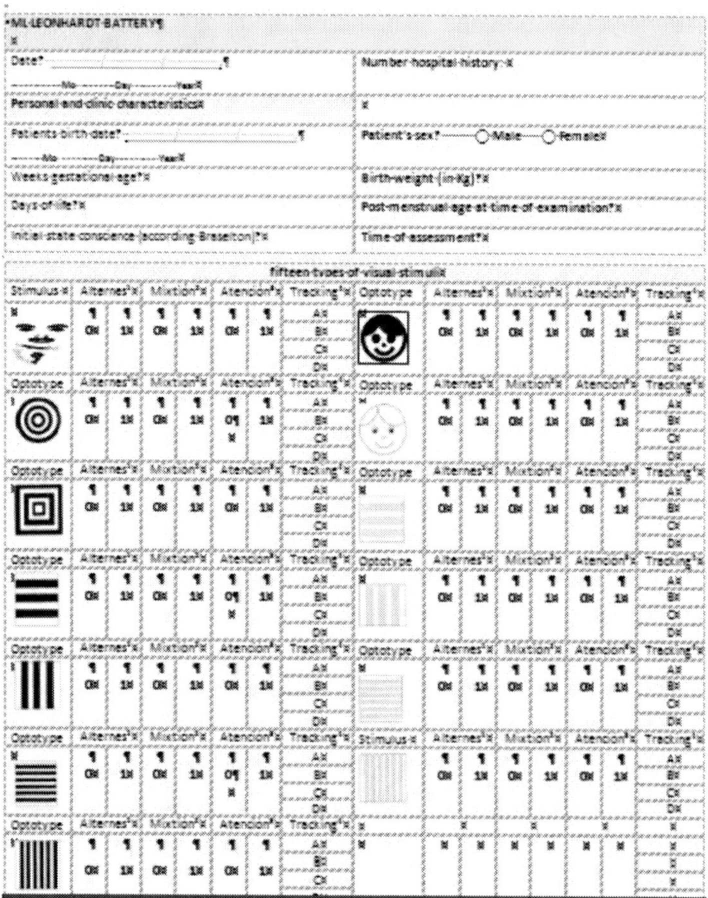

ML LEONHARDT BATTERY

| Date: ___ /___ /___ Mo Day Year | Number hospital history: |
|---|---|
| Personal and clinic characteristics | |
| Patients birth date: ___ /___ /___ Mo Day Year | Patient's sex: ○ Male ○ Female |
| Weeks gestational age: | Birth weight (in Kg): |
| Days of life: | Post-menstrual age at time of examination: |
| Initial state conscience (according Braselton): | Time of assessment: |

fifteen types of visual stimuli

| Stimulus | Alternes[1] | | Mixtion[2] | | Atencion[3] | | Tracking[4] | Optotype | Alternes[1] | | Mixtion[2] | | Atencion[3] | | Tracking[4] |
|---|---|---|---|---|---|---|---|---|---|---|---|---|---|---|---|
| | 0 | 1 | 0 | 1 | 0 | 1 | A B C D | | 0 | 1 | 0 | 1 | 0 | 1 | A B C D |
| **Optotype** | **Alternes[1]** | | **Mixtion[2]** | | **Atencion[3]** | | **Tracking[4]** | **Optotype** | **Alternes[1]** | | **Mixtion[2]** | | **Atencion[3]** | | **Tracking[4]** |
| | 0 | 1 | 0 | 1 | 0 | 1 | A B C D | | 0 | 1 | 0 | 1 | 0 | 1 | A B C D |
| **Optotype** | **Alternes[1]** | | **Mixtion[2]** | | **Atencion[3]** | | **Tracking[4]** | **Optotype** | **Alternes[1]** | | **Mixtion[2]** | | **Atencion[3]** | | **Tracking[4]** |
| | 0 | 1 | 0 | 1 | 0 | 1 | A B C D | | 0 | 1 | 0 | 1 | 0 | 1 | A B C D |
| **Optotype** | **Alternes[1]** | | **Mixtion[2]** | | **Atencion[3]** | | **Tracking[4]** | **Optotype** | **Alternes[1]** | | **Mixtion[2]** | | **Atencion[3]** | | **Tracking[4]** |
| | 0 | 1 | 0 | 1 | 0 | 1 | A B C D | | 0 | 1 | 0 | 1 | 0 | 1 | A B C D |
| **Optotype** | **Alternes[1]** | | **Mixtion[2]** | | **Atencion[3]** | | **Tracking[4]** | **Optotype** | **Alternes[1]** | | **Mixtion[2]** | | **Atencion[3]** | | **Tracking[4]** |
| | 0 | 1 | 0 | 1 | 0 | 1 | A B C D | | 0 | 1 | 0 | 1 | 0 | 1 | A B C D |
| **Optotype** | **Alternes[1]** | | **Mixtion[2]** | | **Atencion[3]** | | **Tracking[4]** | **Stimulus** | **Alternes[1]** | | **Mixtion[2]** | | **Atencion[3]** | | **Tracking[4]** |
| | 0 | 1 | 0 | 1 | 0 | 1 | A B C D | | 0 | 1 | 0 | 1 | 0 | 1 | A B C D |
| **Optotype** | **Alternes[1]** | | **Mixtion[2]** | | **Atencion[3]** | | **Tracking[4]** | | | | | | | | |
| | 0 | 1 | 0 | 1 | 0 | 1 | A B C | | | | | | | | |

CODIGN: [1]Alertness: infant minimum responses to the presentation of the stimulus, showing that he/she is aware and realizes that something is there. Coded: 0 (absent) 1 (present),

[2]Fixation: infant detects and focalizes mono or binoculary on the stimulus, showing some adjustments to the stimulus Coded: 0 (absent) 1 (present)

[3]Attention: infant focuses on the stimuli during a minimum of 3 seconds. Coded: 0 (absent) 1 (present)

[4]Tracking: infant turned his/her eyes (or eye), or both the head and eyes towards a moving stimulus. Coded: A (absent), B (brief -tracking the object is characterized by discontinuous glances-), C (incomplete -continuous movement along the object with the eyes-), and D (complete -continuous tracking of the object with eyes and head-).

Figures 1. Register Proforma of visuals functions with ML Leonhardt Optotype Optotapy Battery.

In this condition the baby is alert and motor activity is minimal. If signs of stress appear during the test application, a small break is taken to allow the child to recover before continuing. In the case of visible signs of stress, the baby is consoled, see table 2 and 3.

*Position and environment:* The baby may be held in the arms of their parents or staff or in a crib. When the battery has to be applied in the incubator, the evaluator holds the baby with one hand while presenting the stimulus with the other, allowing the child to move freely. Light and environmental noise are carefully controlled: ambient light should be low and the atmosphere should be calm, quiet and relaxed.

*Presentation of the optotypes and eliciting responses:* The optotypes are displayed consecutively to the baby, one at a time, in front of their eyes at a distance of between 14 and 20 cm. Each stimulus is presented with slight movements in the same spatial axis, in order to keep the baby's attention. The examiner remains outside the line of vision and avoids talking to the infants. Having attracted the baby's attention to the stimulus, the examiner will attempt to fix and maintain attention to the stimulus during the three seconds required. The examiner tries to elicit the tracking response to the visual optotypes. The application therefore requires appropriate training.

*Application time:* Administration time is between 10 and 15 minutes. The test is usually applied in a single session, but pauses may be needed to elicit optimal performance from the newborn.

**Table 3. Consoling strategies**

| Consoling strategies |
|---|
| Speaking softly to the baby |
| Gently touching the feet, hands, chin |
| Waiting for the baby's response |
| Containment of his body |
| When the baby is quiet and vital signs are stable the ML Leonhardt battery can be applied |
| Breaks in case of fatigue |
| Recovering attention |

## Register Proforma

The responses are recorded on a Proforma Register, see figure 1.

## Psychometric Properties

The test-retest reliability of ML Leonhardt Battery was analyzed using the inter-observer Kappa coefficient in a sample of 20 full-term newborns. Observers were two neonatal specialists experienced in the use of the battery. The instrument was applied between three and 48 hours after birth. A mean kappa coefficient of .94 was obtained; depending on the visual behaviors and optotypes analyzed, kappa values ranged between .80 and 1.00, thus indicating good reliability.

## 3.1. Studies Conducted with Battery Ml Leonhardt

### *3.1.1. Term and Preterm Newborns*

Between 2006-08, several studies [20, 21] were conducted to assess the visual capacity of preterm and term infants. The objectives were to contrast the visual function of term and preterm infants and to analyze the discriminative ability of high- and low-contrast optotypes in preterm newborns. The control group comprised 50 infants (60.5% boys and 39.5% girls) born at term. The mean time of gestation was 39 weeks (SD = 1.2) and birth weight was 3.366 (SD = 0.5). The test's mean application time was 13.7 minutes. The test was completed in 67.4% of cases; in the remaining 32.6% the main reason for non-completion was sleep.

The preterm low risk group comprised 100 infants (54% boys and 46% girls). The mean time of gestation was 29.7 (SD = 2.6), birth weight was 1.287 (SD = 0.45), and at the time of application of the test the mean weight was 1.898 (SD = 0.60), seeking the clinical stability of the child. The mean application time of the test was 7.8 minutes; 50% completed the test. Seventy-five per cent of babies were applied the test in the order of presentation described in the optotype protocol, while the remaining 25% began the test with low-contrast optotypes.

The aim was to analyse the discriminative ability of high- and low-contrast optotypes in this group of infants. The studies provided information on the visual behavioral responses of alertness, fixation, attention and tracking in term and preterm newborns, and on the ability to discriminate between high and low contrast optotypes in preterm infants.

a) Visual behavioral responses of alertness, fixation, attention and tracking in term and preterm newborns

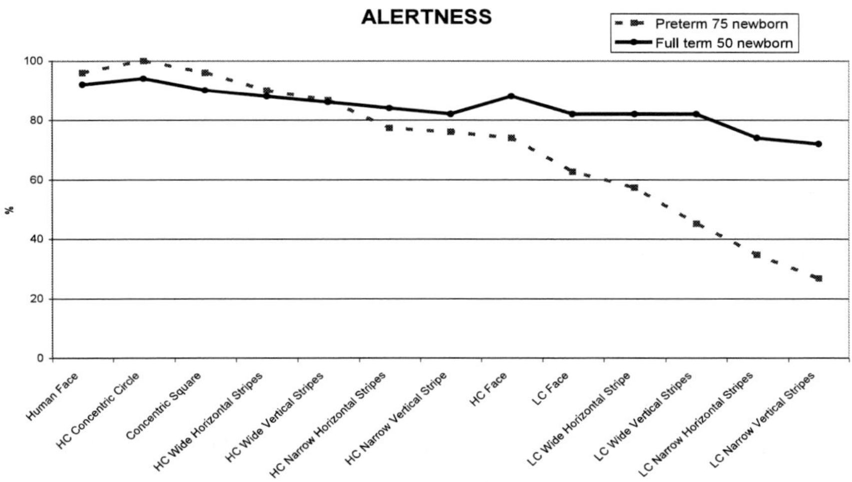


Figure 2. Visual behavioral responses of alertness in term and preterm newborns.Visual Functions: Alertness.

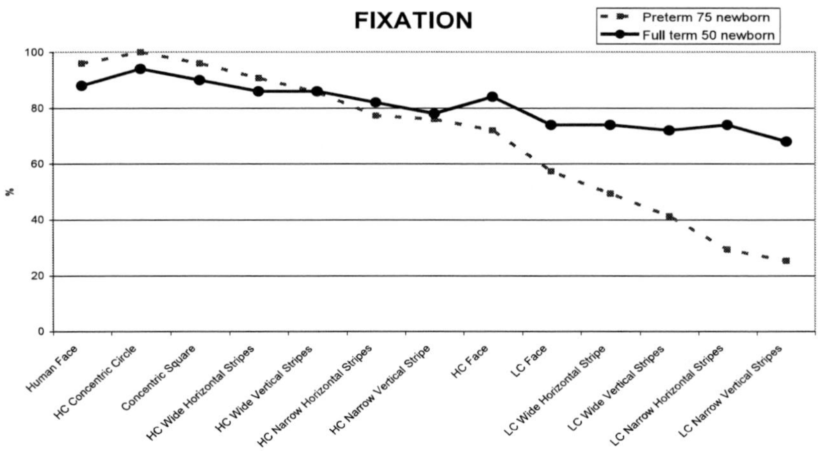


Figure 3. Visual behavioral responses of fixation in term and preterm newborns.

Almost all the term newborns showed alert behavior towards high-contrast (between 82% and 94%) and low-contrast optotypes (between 72% to 82%). The preterm group showed alert behavior toward high-contrast optotypes (between 74% and 100%) but when low-contrast optotypes were introduced a progressive decline in their response was observed (between 26.7% and 62.7%), see figure 2.

## Visual Functions: Fixation

Most term newborns displayed fixation behavior towards high-contrast (between 78% and 94%) and low-contrast optotypes (between 68% and 74%). The preterm group showed fixation behavior toward high-contrast optotypes (between 72% and 100%) but when low-contrast optotypes were introduced a progressive decline in their response was observed (between 25.3% and 57.3%), see figure 3.

## Visual Functions: Attention

Most term newborn showed attention behavior towards the high-contrast optotypes (between 78% and 90%) and low-contrast (between 62% and 70%).

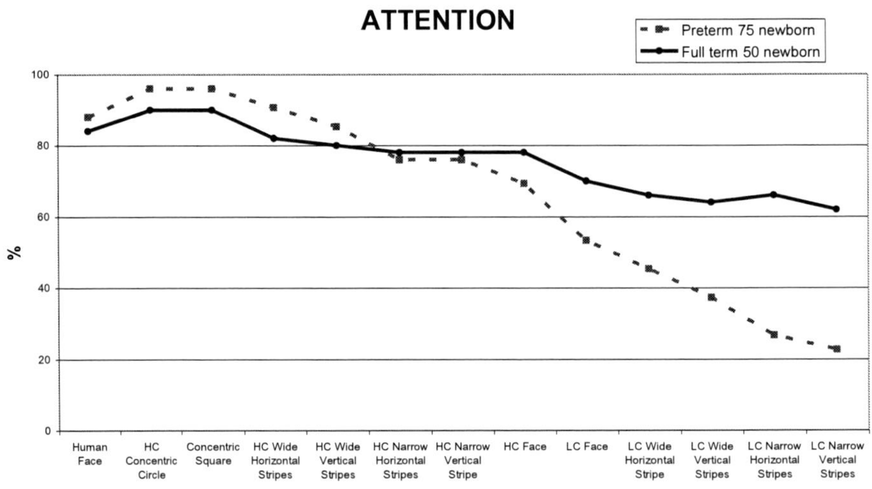


Figure 4. Visual behavioral responses of attention in term and preterm newborns.

The preterm group showed attention behavior towards high-contrast optotypes (between 69.3% and 96%) but when low-contrast optotypes were introduced a progressive decline in their response was observed (between 22.7% and 53.3%), see figure 4.

Since low-contrast optotypes require more effort in the visual response from the baby, it was interpreted that the decline observed in the preterm group in the three visual behaviors analysed (alertness, attention, and fixation) was probably a manifestation of visual fatigue.

## Visual Functions: Tracking

The percentage of term newborns who were able to perform complete tracking with face and eyes for each optotype ranged between 20% and 34% for high-contrast and between 6% and 16% for low-contrast. There was a decrease in complete tracking when low-contrast optotypes were displayed. The preterm newborns showed complete tracking behavior towards high-contrast optotypes (between 13.3% to 22.7%), but when low-contrast optotypes were introduced a decline in their responses was observed (between 5.3% and 6.3%), see figure 5.

A quarter of preterm infants performed visual tracking behaviors. The tracking percentages are somewhat lower in the preterm group. In both groups there was a decrease in visual tracking behavior in low-contrast optotypes, but term infants could not recover it.

This was interpreted as increased resilience of the visual response of term infants compared to preterm infants.

b) Discriminative ability of high and low contrast optotypes in preterm infants

Infants showed better visual responses to high-contrast than to low-contrast optotypes, which was attributed to their growing weariness during the application of the test.

However, it is unclear whether the decline in performance was due to fatigue or to the acuity of the optotypes. To examine this point, 25 preterm newborns were administered first the low-contrast optotypes from the battery. Figure 6 shows the three application conditions: a) start with high-contrast optotypes, b) continue implementation with low-contrast optotypes (75 preterm newborns) and c) start with low-contrast optotypes (25 preterm newborns) in visual fixation behaviour, figure 6.

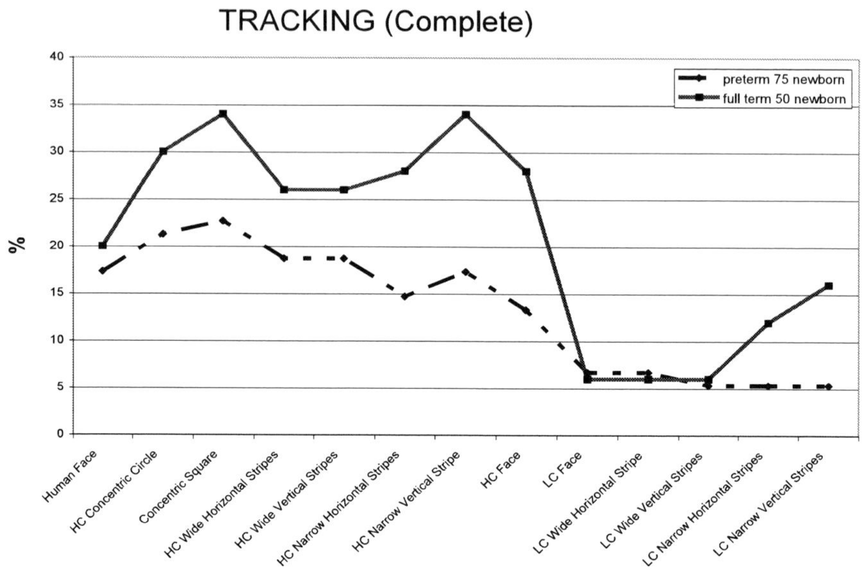


Figure 5. Visual behavioral responses of complete tracking in term and preterm newborns.

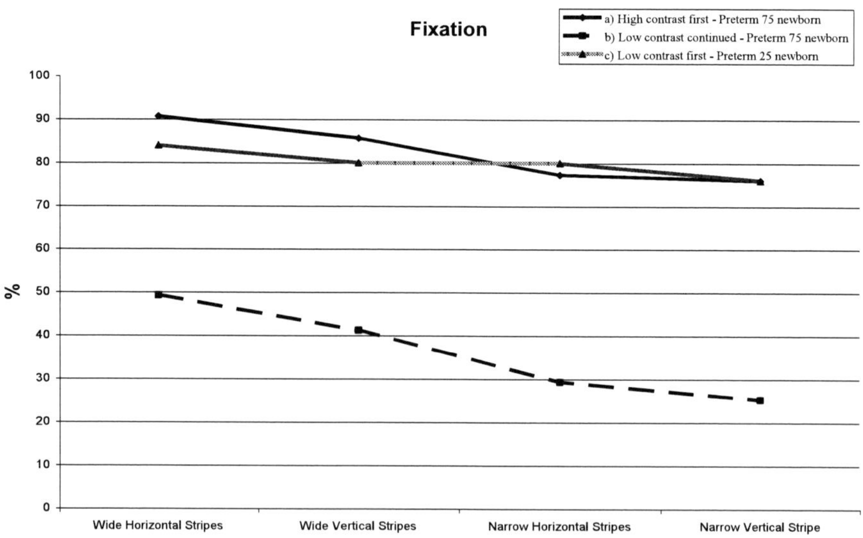


Figure 6. Discriminative ability of visual fixation behavior of optotypes high-and-low contrast in preterm newborn.

## Visual Functions: Fixation

The preterm newborns showed fixation behavior towards the high-contrast optotypes (between 76% and 91%, condition a), but when low-contrast optotypes were introduced (condition b) a progressive decline in their responses was observed, ranging between 25.3% and 49.3%. The preterm group that started with low-contrast optotypes (condition c) showed a fixation behavior of between 76% and 84%, figure 7. The success rates in conditions a) and c) are comparable, suggesting that the fixation response among preterm infants is similar when the application starts with either a high or a low contrast optotype. In condition b, in which the low-contrast optotypes were applied after the high-contrast, the visual fixation behavior decreased. In conclusion, the decrease in visual behavior of infants with low-contrast optotypes after previous exposure to high-contrast optotypes is due to fatigue and not to the acuity of the optotypes. This confirms our initial hypothesis.

### *3.1.2. Preterm Newborns with and without Brain Injury*

Recently, Leonhardt et al. [3] analyzed the differences in visual function between preterm newborns with and without brain injury, using the ML Leonhardt Optotype Battery. They compare infants' visual abilities related to alertness, fixation, attention and tracking.

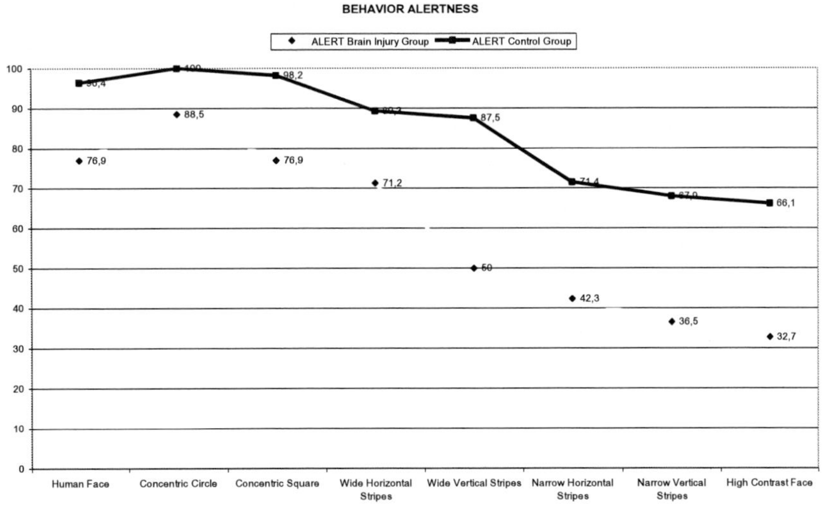


Figure 7. Visual behavioral responses of alertness in newborn preterm with and without brain injury.

## Subjects

All preterm infants were recruited via the Neonatal Intensive Care Units (NICU) of three maternity hospitals in Barcelona, Spain. *Control group* (CG, without brain injury) comprised 56 infants (51.8% boys and 48.2% girls). 45.2% were considered to be at high risk (GA < 33 weeks and GA < 33 weeks and weight < 1.500 kg), and 54.7% at moderate risk (GA ≥ 34 weeks and weight ≥ 1.501 kg). All infants included had a normal retinal condition. Forty per cent completed the test in the mean application time of 7.8 minutes (SD = 3.6), while 60% did not complete it, due mainly to sleep. The *Brain Injury group* (BIG) comprised 48 infants (52.1% boys and 47.9% girls). 46.3% were considered to be at high risk (GA < 33 weeks and w GA < 33 weeks and weight < 1.500 kg), and 53.6% at moderate risk (GA ≥ 34 weeks and weight ≥ 1.501 kg). All preterm infants were evaluated at 72 hours (SD = 5) with cranial ultrasound scan, and those suspected of having brain injury underwent neonatal serial brain MRI and neurological examination by the team of neurologists at each hospital. The mean application time was 10 minutes (SD = 4.5); six per cent completed the test, while 94% did not due mainly to sleep.

## Instrument

The ML Leonhardt battery was applied by the author of the test in all groups. Visual behavioral responses of alertness, fixation, attention and tracking of the 15 optotypes were analyzed. The infants were propped up at 30º in a supine position in a quiet environment with dimmed background lighting to facilitate eye-opening, and with few stimuli in the surroundings. The examiner avoided talking to the baby while presenting the visual stimuli. The optotypes were moved slowly in order to keep the child's attention. The children were in a state of consciousness of 4 or 5 during examination [22]. The battery was applied in a single session but short breaks were introduced to elicit the best response. If the baby was not able to complete the test, the test was not repeated.

## Statistical Analysis

The statistical analysis included a descriptive analysis of the characteristics of sex, birth-weight, gestational age, days of life and postmenstrual age at time of examination. Chi-squared or Mann Whitney U tests were used to compare these variables in the brain injury and control groups. The visual function behaviors related to alertness, fixation and attention were analyzed according to the percentage differences between the two groups for each stimulus. Differences in tracking behavior between the groups were analyzed for each stimulus by means of the chi-squared test. The level of significance was set at $p < 0.005$. All data were analyzed using SPSS® (version 16.0) for Windows.

## Results

Low-risk preterm infants showed better responses for the visual functions of alertness, fixation, attention and tracking than preterm infants in the brain injury group.

More than 90% of the low-risk preterm infants looked at the *human face.* However, when a human face was presented in a two-dimensional drawing after other optotypes, the observed outcomes were less successful than when a real human face was presented, in the control group and especially in the brain injury group (BIG). We suggest that brain injured infants are unlikely to be attracted by the stimulus (due to the complexity of the pattern) or to maintain attention, with fatigue appearing very quickly (with only about 4-6 minutes elapsing between the presentation of the human face and the high-contrast face drawing).

With regard to the *concentric stimulus (circle and square)*, low-risk preterm infants of 36.4 weeks PMA had a success rate > 96% with these optotypes with a spatial frequency of 0.50 cycles per degree, in visual alertness, fixation and attention responses. The brain injury preterm infants of 40 weeks PMA showed less mature responses than the control group in the visual behavior analyzed – attention responses – in which their success rates were about 65%. The percentages differences in success between the CG and the BIG on concentric forms become progressively more pronounced. Our results for the low-risk preterm group corroborate those of Ricci [18, 21], who found that over 91% of low-risk preterm infants showed stable fixation at 35 weeks PMA, rising to 97% at 40 weeks, see figure 8 and 9.

With regard to the *wide stripes of 0.25 cycles per degree* (horizontal and vertical) we found levels of success in alertness, fixation and attention behaviors of between 80% and 89% in low-risk preterm infants of 40 weeks PMA.

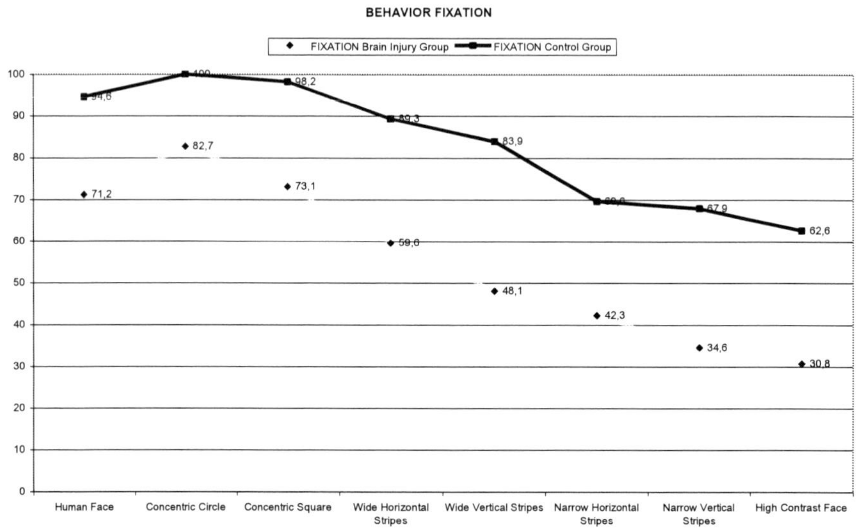


Figure 8. Visual behavioral responses of fixation in newborn preterm with and without brain injury.

When this stripe stimulus increased in spatial frequency up to 0.50 cycles per degree, the level of success decreased. The difference in the percentage success rate between the BIG and CG in these visual behaviors was around 30%.

This finding of lower visual ability in the BIG on all the stimuli presented may reflect difficulties in subcortical maturation, and may also be due to associated pathologies or impairment in other brain systems. Ricci et al.[22] indicated that visual abnormalities were higher in preterm infants with brain lesions, specifically in those with PVL.

As regards *tracking behavior*, the low-risk preterm infants showed a very different pattern of responses to the brain injury group, in which the category of "absent" (child did not turn his/her eyes (or eye), or both the head and eyes towards a moving stimulus) was the predominant response (see figure X). When considering complete tracking responses (continuous tracking of the object with the eyes, at an angle of between 30 and 90 degrees), the range of success in the BIG did not differ greatly from the control group – between 10% and 20% depending on the optotype. Our study found a much poorer performance in the BIG than Ricci [32].

The circle and square of .50 cycles per degree obtained better success rates than the wider horizontal and vertical striped figures (.25 cycles per degree) which one would expect to capture better the children's attention.

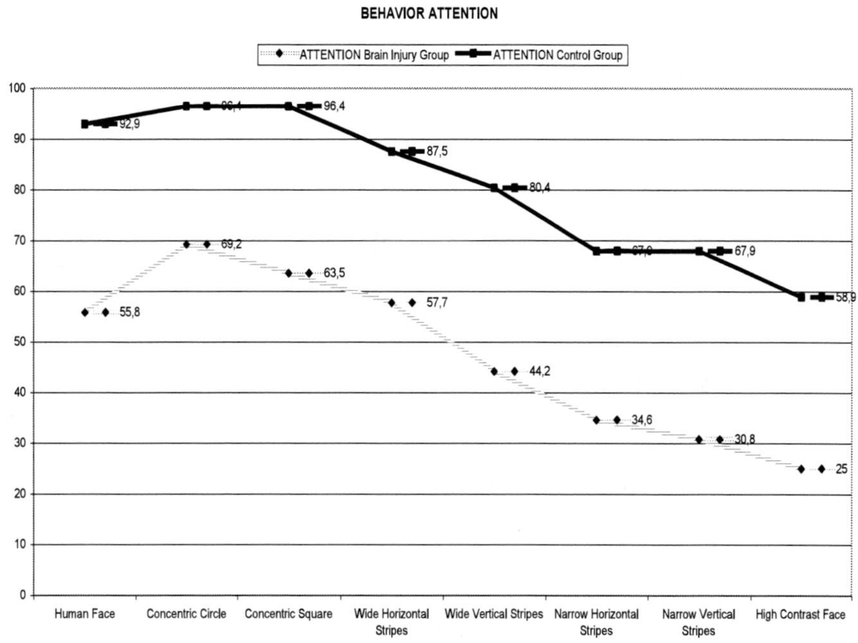


Figure 9. Visual behavioral responses of attention in newborn preterm with and without brain injury.Those authors indicated that 97% of preterm newborns at 35 weeks PMA and 100% at 40 weeks PMA showed accentuated maturation in terms of discriminating striped black/white targets of spatial frequencies of at least 0.64 cycles per degree. Our low-risk preterm group presented poorer results, although the test card used is somewhat broader (0.50 c/degree) than the ones used in Ricci's studies. In addition, less than half of the brain injury group attained good visual performance, thus indicating notable difficulties in visual function. Our data should be reanalyzed in more homogeneous groups, specifically in infants with different kinds of brain injury. At present, it is difficult to distinguish between the effects of subcortical impairment, attention impairment, and the fatigue that appears during the application of the test.

The difference in performance does not seem to be linked only to the spatial frequency of cycles per degree. We should study the influence of the Gestalt concept of "good form", as a process of perception at these early ages.

In conclusion, it would be beneficial to promote early stimulation of visual function in all infants who present difficulties. Not only the optical functions should be assessed but also the ventral visual pathways, which are linked to the identification and selection of objects, and the dorsal pathways, which are linked to the systems of movement, space and action [24].

Our findings differ from those of other researchers such as Ricci et al. [14,16] with regard to the narrow horizontal and vertical stripe stimulus.

We conclude that brain injured infants show visual difficulties that can be identified in the first weeks of their life. This highlights the importance of early intervention with this population in order to improve both visual functions and attention behavior [5, 14, 26].

## CONCLUSION

At present, there are still doubts about whether newborns can see. There are many parents who think that their children do not look at them, or cannot see their faces. This belief has been fuelled for a long time by a lack of appropriate instruments able to assess the vision of infants, especially of preterm infants. The ML Leonhardt Optotype Battery is an easy to apply instrument that can inform about visual functions from the beginning of life.

When parents look at their child and identify the receptivity of their infant's gaze, they strengthen this receptivity and encourage the infant to establish visual contact again and again. This reinforces the manifestations of attachment and therefore forges the affective link at an early stage.

Newborns have several visual abilities from the moment they open their eyes. The studies and the assessment batteries of visual functioning we have described in this chapter verify that visual functioning is acquired very early in life.

Infants can look at the faces of their parents and caregivers. The face is the most potent stimulus to attract their gaze. Our studies show that both preterm and term newborns presented with high-contrast optotypes of different shapes and different spatial frequencies horizontally, vertically and in an arc can display alertness, fixation, attention and visual tracking. Visual attention, in general, can be held for a few seconds if the object is at a distance of 20-30 cm.

Children with brain lesions present a significant delay in the beginning of the development of visual functions. When they explore optotypes visible signs of stress and behavioral fatigue may appear that oblige them to withdraw their attention from the external stimulus.

The studies presented in this chapter aim to assess infants' visual capabilities and to detect visual impairments related to neurological injury or delayed maturation. As Atkinson notes, "a wide range of behavioral and cognitive functions in the developing child are linked to vision" [12]. An understanding of the visual functions of newborn is of particular interest not only in the area of sensorial impairment, but also in the area of future behavioral and cognitive impairment of the functions linked to visual abilities.

It is very important to identify children's visual difficulties and visual needs in the first week or first months of life, in order to apply early intervention programs. These programs will benefit the infant's general development, allowing the establishment of a better emotional link with their parents and improving the development of cognitive aspects that are linked to visual maturation, such as visual perception or visual coordination. The early implementation of these stimulation programs can achieve a better start to life for these children.

## REFERENCES


[1] Dubois J, Hertz-Pannier L, Dehaene-Lambertz G, Cointepas Y, Le Bihan D. Assessment of the early organization and maturation of infants' cerebral white matter fiber bundles: a feasibility study using quantitative diffusion tensor imaging and tractography. *Neuroimage,* 2006; 3 (4): 1121 – 32.

[2] Ricci D, Cesarini L, Groppo M, De Carli A, Gallini F, Serrao F, Fumagalli M, Cowan F, Ramenghi LA, Anker S, Mercuri E, Mosca F. Early assessment of visual function in full term newborns. *Early Hum. Dev.,* 2008; 84 (2): 107-13.

[3] Leonhardt M, Forns M, Calderón C, Reinoso M, Gargallo E. Visual performance in preterm infants with brain injuries compared with healthy preterm infants. *Early Hum. Dev.,* 2012; 88 (8): 669-675.

[4] Amiel-Tison C. Update of the Amiel-Tison neurologic assessment for the term neonate or at 40 weeks corrected age. *Pediatr. Neurol.,* 2002; 27 (3): 196-212.

[5] Brazelton TB, Nugent K. *Neonatal Behavioural Assessment Scale*, 3rd Edition. London: Mac Keith Press; 1995.

[6] Fazzi E, Signorini SG, Bova SM, La Piana R, Ondei P, Bertone C, Misefari W, Bianchi PE. Spectrum of visual disorders in children with cerebral visual impairment. *J. Child Neurol.,* 2007; 22 (3): 294-301.

[7] Mercuri E, Baranello G, Romeo DM, Cesarini L, Ricci D. The development of vision. *Early Hum. Dev.,* 2007; 83 (12): 795-800.

[8] Guzzetta A, Mercuri E, Cioni G. Visual disorders in children with brain lesion 2: Visual impairment associated with cerebral palsy. *Eur. J. Paediatric. Neurol.,* 2001; 5 (3): 115-19.

[9] Ramenghi LA, Rutherford M, Fumagalli M, Bassi L, Messner H, Counsell S, Mosca F. Neonatal neuroimaging: going beyond the pictures. *Early Hum. Dev.,* 2009; 85: S75-7.

[10] Ramenghi LA, Fumagalli M, Bassi L, Groppo M, De Carli A, Fanaro S, Mosca F. Brain Maturation of Preterm Newborn Babies: New Insights. *J. Pediatr. Gastroenterol. Nutr.,* 2007; 45: S143-6.

[11] Kato T, Watanabe K. Visual evoked potential in the newborn: Does it have predictive value? *Semin in Fetal and Neonatal Med.,* 2006; 11 (6): 459-63.

[12] Atkinson J, Anker S, Rae S, Hughes C, Braddick O. A test battery of child development for examining functional vision (ABCDEFV). *Strabismus,* 2002; 10 (4): 245-69.

[13] Guzzetta A, Cioni G, Cowan F, Mercuri E. Visual Disorders in Children with brain lesions: 1. Maturation on visual function in infants with neonatal brain lesions: correlation with neuroimaging. *Eur. J. Paediatr. Neurol.,* 2001; 5 (3): 107- 14.

[14] Ricci D, Romeo DM, Serrao F, Gallini F, Leone D, Longo M, Albamonte E, Romeo MG, Mazzone D, Romagnoli C, Cowan F, Mercuri E. Early assessment of visual function in preterm infats: how early is early? *Early Hum. Dev.,* 2010, 86 (1): 29-33.

[15] Ricci D, Romeo DM, Serrao F, Cesarini L, Gallini F, Cota F, Leone D, Zuppa AA, Romagnoli C, Cowan F, Mercuri E. Application of a neonatal assessment of visual function in a population of low risk full-term newborn. *Early Hum. Dev.,* 2008; 84 (4): 277-80.

[16] Ricci D, Cesarini L, Romeo DM, Gallini F, Serrao F, Groppo M, De Carli A, Cota F, Lepore D, Molle F, Ratiglia R, De Carolis MP, Mosca F, Romagnoli C, Guzzetta F, Cowan F, Ramenghi LA, Mercuri E. Visual Function at 35 and 40 weeks' postmenstrual age in low-risk preterm infants. *Pediatrics,* 2008; 122 (6): e1193-98.

[17] Ricci D, Cesarini L, Gallini F, Serrao F, Leone D, Baranello G, Cota F, Pane M, Brogna C, De Rose P, Vasco G, Alfieri P, Staccioli S, Romeo DM, Tinelli F, Molle F, Lepore D, Baldascino A, Ramenghi LA, Torrioli MG, Romagnoli C, Cowan F, Atkinson J, Cioni G, Mercuri E. Cortical visual function in preterm infants in the first year. *J. Pediatr.,* 2010; 156 (4): 550-5.

[18] Atkinson J. The developing visual brain. England: Oxford University Press; 2000.

[19] Leonhardt M. Detección de respuestas visuales en recién nacidos pretérmino: resultados preliminares de un estudio piloto con batería de optotipos. *Revista Integración, sobre ceguera y deficiencia visual,* 2007: 51; 7-19.

[20] Leonhardt M. Primera intervención en hospitales. Atención a diferentes poblaciones en las primeras edades. Perspectivas de futuro. In: A Lafuente (ed). *Construir juntos espacios de esperanza*. Madrid: ONCE, 2008.

[21] Leonhardt M. Valoración de la capacidad visual en recién nacidos pretérmino de bajo riesgo. *Revista de Atención Temprana,* 2006: 9 (2); 65-73.

[22] Brazelton TB, Nugent K. Escala para la evaluación del comportamiento neonatal. Barcelona: Paidós, 1995.

[23] Brazelton, T. B. Neonatal Behavioral Assessment Scale. Clinics in Developmental Medicine, No. 50, London: William Heinemann Medical Books. Philadelphia: J. B. Lippincott, 1973.

[24] Ricci D, Romeo DM, Gallini F, Groppo M, Cesarini L, Pisoni S, Serrao F, Papacci P, Contaldo I, Perrino F, Brogna C, Bianco F, Baranello G, Sacco A, Quintiliani M, Ometto A, Cilauro S, Mosca F, Romagnoli C, Romeo MG, Cowan F, Cioni G, Ramenghi L, Mercuri E. Early visual assessment in preterm infants with and without brain lesions: correlation with visual and neurodevelopmental outcome at 12 months. *Early Hum. Dev.,* 2011; 87 (3): 177-82.

[25] Fowles ER. The Brazelton Neonatal Behavioral Assessment Scale and maternal identity. *AMC AM J. Matern. Child Nurs.,* 1999; 24: 287-93.

[26] Ramenghi LA, Ricci D, Mercuri E, Groppo M, De Carli A, Ometto A, Fumagalli M, Bassi L, Pisoni S, Cioni G, Mosca F. Visual performance and brain structures in the developing brain of pre-term infants. *Early Hum. Dev.,* 2010: 86 Supp 1:73-5.

[27] Leonhardt M., Un estudio sobre la valoración de la capacidad visual en recién nacidos pretérmino de riesgo, *La revista de l'ACAP,* 2008; 29: 8-30.

[28] Leonhardt M. Optotipos "ML" Leonhardt para neonatos y niños con discapacidad. La evaluación Visual en atención temprana, Fund. Ramon Martí Bonet, Barcelona, 2012

[29] Teller DY, McDonald MA, Preston K, Sebris SL, Dobson V. Assessment of visual acuity in infants and children: the acuity card procedure. *Dev. Med. Child Neurol.,* 1986; 28 (6): 779-89.
[30] Hyvärinen L, Näsänen R. Laurinen P. New visual acuity test for preschool children. *Acta. Ophthalmol. (Copenh),* 1980; 58: 507-11.
[31] Bailey IL, Lovie JE. New design principles for visual acuity letter charts. *Am. J. Optom. Physiol. Opt., 1976;* 53: 740-45.
[32] Ricci D, Cesarini L, Groppo M, De Carli A, Gallini F, Serrao F, Fumnagalli M, Cowan F, Ramenghi L, Anker S, Mercuri E, Mosca F. Early assessment of visual function in fullterm newborns. *Early Hum. Dev.,* 2008; 84: 107-13.

In: Screening Tests
Editor: Marguerite Gauthier
ISBN: 978-1-62417-963-1
© 2013 Nova Science Publishers, Inc.

*Chapter 3*

# NAILFOLD CAPILLAROSCOPY: A BASIC SCREENING TOOL IN RAYNAUD'S PHENOMENON

***Athina Pyrpasopoulou*** * ***and Spyros Aslanidis***
Hippokration General Hospital, Thessaloniki, Greece

## ABSTRACT

The term "Raynaud's phenomenon" refers to a defined triphasic colour change pattern (white, blue, red) of the skin of the fingers. The initial pallor, which may lead to cyanosis (blue coloration) of the digits, is followed by reactive hyperemia and can be accompanied by numbness, paresthesias and pain. Raynaud's is triggered by exposure to cold, emotional stress and specific drugs. Pathophysiologically it is characterized by an excessive vasoconstrictive response (dominance of vasoconstrisctive over vasodilatory factors) of the small arterioles and the digital arteries.

Etiologically it can be classified as primary or secondary, mainly either to systemic sclerosis and related diseases, or to the thoracic outlet syndrome. As such, Raynaud's phenomenon represents an important clinical manifestation of microvascular involvement. Rare cases of

* Address correspondence to: Dr Athina Pyrpasopoulou, PhD, 2nd Propedeutic Dept of Internal Medicine, Hippokration General Hospital, Konstantinoupoleos 49, 54643, Thessaloniki, Greece. Tel: +302310892072. Fax: +302310892117. E-mail: a.pyrpasopoulou@ doctors. org.uk.

paraneoplastic Raynaud's have been described, the pathogenesis of which remains unclarified, has however been most likely attributed to neuroendocrine substances secreted by the tumor.

Despite the evolution of the technology involved over the decades, nailfold capillaroscopy remains very simple in principle. The term refers to the non-invasive observation of the nailfold capillary bed. Nailfold capillaroscopy can be performed with basic equipment such as a magnifying lens, an ophthalmoscope, a dermatoscope/ stereomicroscope or a conventional wide field microscope; the nailfold video capillaroscope, however, is the gold standard tool, and provides the technology for the visualization and analysis both of morphological as well as rheological parameters of the skin microvasculature. Qualitative and quantitative microangiopathic parameters that can be recorded and analyzed include, among others, microhemorrhages, plexus morphology, capillary density, and morphologic anomalies of the end row loops.

In normal conditions, or in primary Raynaud's, the normal nailfold capillaroscopic pattern shows a regular disposition of the capillary loops along with the nailbed. In subjects suffering from secondary Raynaud's phenomenon, alterations of the capillaroscopic findings should alert the physician of the possibility of a connective tissue disease or other conditions not yet detected.

This review aims to outline the major characteristics of the normal nailfold microvascular network and the healthy variations that may be encountered in relation to age, race, employment etc, and highlight its applicability not only as a powerful tool in the screening of a variety of vascular disorders, in particular of autoimmune origin, but also as a potent tool in the follow-up of patients with established microvascular disorders in response to treatment.

As microcirculation involvement is attracting increasing interest in chronic vascular diseases such as diabetes mellitus or hypertension, as a prognostic marker for macrovascular disease and target organ involvement, the acquaintance with and application of techniques assessing microvascular compromise gains particular significance. The advantages of capillaroscopy (low cost, uninvasiveness, repeatability, high sensitivity, good specificity and easy interpretation of the results) render this technique a valuable asset for the clinician.

## Pathophysiology of Raynaud's Phenomenon

The term Raynaud's phenomenon has been appointed to the discoloration of the fingers. Typical Raynaud's, as first described by Maurice Raynaud in 1862, is characterized by the triphasic color change of the fingers (white in the decreased blood perfusion initial phase, blue in the hypoxic cyanotic phase and , finally, red in the reperfusion phase) accompanied by a sense of fullness or tautness, which may be painful [1]. Digital involvement is not uniform; the thumb is significantly less frequently involved [2]. The phenomenon is paroxysmal, usually lasting no more than half an hour; it can however persist for hours. The recurrent microvasculature vasospasm, whose effect is obvious in the fingers, can also affect other areas of the body (toes, ears, nose, tongue etc), as well as internal organs. Triggers are cold, emotional stress, drugs/ chemicals and physical factors. When associated with an underlying disorder Raynaud's phenomenon is termed Raynaud's syndrome.

Raynaud's phenomenon is thought to be related to vasospasm (imbalance between vasoconstricting and vasodilating factors). Under normal conditions, the vascular tone is controlled by complex interactions between the endothelium, the muscular layer, and autonomic and sensory nerves that innevate the vessels and a number of soluble mediators. Vasoconstricting substances such as catecholamines, endothelin 1, and 5-hydroxytryptamine, which may be released in response to cold exposure, may cause digital artery closure and the associated symptoms of Raynaud's phenomenon. In some cases, especially when there is an associated underlying autoimmune disease, neutrophils and platelets are activated, with resultant release of inflammatory cytokines, which contribute to endothelial damage seen in more severe secondary Raynaud's syndrome [3]. Besides the direct effect of vasoconsticting substances on alpha adrenergic receptors of the vascular smooth muscle, hyper-reactivity of the sympathetic nervous system has been described as a prominent feature of the pathogenesis of Raynaud's phenomenon. Morever, neuropeptides released from nerve endings such as calcitonin gene related peptide or substance P may additionally contribute to the abnormal vasospastic response [4].

Raynaud's phenomenon is four times more common in women than men, appearing on average at the age of 40, [5]. Indeed, basal cutaneous flow in the hands and fingers of young women appears to be decreased when compared to that of men [6]. This effect could be associated with an increase in the sympathetically induced vascular tone in women and may be mediated by the action of oestrogens on responses generated by $\alpha$ adrenoreceptors [7, 8]. However, when normally menstruating women were tested under a similar protocol during the early follicular phase (low hormone state), there was no difference in either the magnitude of vasoconstriction or the individual contributions of sympathetic transmitters compared to the high hormone state induced by oral contraceptives [9]. Aging appears to have a negative effect on reflex cutaneous vasoconstriction; this may be attributed to the dysfunction of several regulatory mechanisms: the sympathetic autonomic nerve signal preceding constriction, impaired transmitter synthesis and release from the axon, and loss of post-junctional end-organ responsiveness [10].

Despite significant progress in the understanding of pathophysiologic mechanisms involved in the pathogenesis of the syndome, the complete deciphering of the phenomenon may have particular significance in several clinical populations including essential hypertensives type 2 diabetics, and CHF patients, who are further at risk from suffering the consequences of attenuated reflex vasodilation due to pathology-, pharmacologic- and primary aged-related impairments in reflex vasodilator mechanisms.

## Epidemiology and Classification of Raynaud's Phenomenon

The prevalence of Raynaud's syndrome is determined by geographic and climatic factors [11], occupation, local living conditions, environmental influences, and genetic factors [5]. A familial predisposition has been recorded in at least 3% of the affected individuals. By demonstrating a higher concordance in MZ twins compared with DZ twins in a UK study with 288 twin pairs, it can be conferred that Raynaud has a genetic basis, with a doubling of risk of the phenomenon in first-degree relatives of affected individuals [12]. In Europe, Raynaud occurs in 5 to 20 % of the population. In North America (US), its incidence ranges between 4% and 11% in women and between 3% and 8% in men [13-16]. In a total of 1540 forestry workers in Quebec, the prevalence of Raynaud's phenomenon was found to be as high as 30.5% among chain-saw users and 8.7% among nonusers [17]. Indeed among a general population cohort in Great Britain of 12907 adults of working age, about one-third of men reporting Raynaud's phenomenon had been exposed to hand-induced vibration [18]. Among other factors besides sex, age, and occupation (exposure to cold/vibration), heavy alcohol consumption, higher psychological burden, and higher diastolic, but not systolic blood pressure, in hypertensives treated with anti-hypertensive medications were found to correlate with the manifestation of Raynaud's phenomenon [19, 20]. Smoking may influence hand–arm vibration syndrome [21]; moreover, it seems to be associated with the severity of Raynaud in patients with underlying vascular disease [22]. However, from a large epidemiological study no association could be established between Raynaud's phenomenon and cigarette consumption [23].

Raynaud is a phenomenon, which can be primary (idiopathic) or secondary to a number of different conditions, mainly rheumatological diseases and a variety of other causes, such as extrinsic vascular obstruction, as in thoracic outlet syndrome, paraproteinaemias and certain drugs/chemicals [24-26]. The ratio of the two conditions lies vastly in favor of primary Raynaud (~4:1). In a clinical sample of 304 and 112 patients with Raynaud respectively, the initial prevalence of secondary Raynaud measured 11-14.3%, with an annual incidence of transition from primary to secondary Raynaud of 1-1.4% [27, 28].

The exact pathogenesis and pathophysiology vary between these conditions. Leroy and Medsger proposed criteria for the classification of primary Raynaud's phenomenon; symmetry of attacks, absence of tissue necrosis, ulceration or gangrene, absence of a secondary cause, negative antinuclear antibodies, normal nailfold capillaroscopy and a normal erythrocyte sedimentation rate [29]. Both primary as well as secondary Raynaud can appear at any age (from the age of very young children to ages older than 80 years, [30]). However, secondary Raynaud usually manifests after the age of 30 years [31]. Secondary Raynaud's phenomenon is associated with painful and asymmetric attacks, ischemic skin lesions, positive autoantibodies, capillaroscopic abnormalities and/or clinical features suggestive of underlying rheumatological conditions. Among the connective tissue diseases associated with Raynaud's phenomenon, systemic sclerosis has the highest frequency; more than 90% of patients with systemic sclerosis exhibit Raynaud's phenomenon [32]. To be able to recognize the cause triggering Raynaud's in a patient, one needs to track down the patient's occupational, smoking and drug history, and to perform a careful physical examination, nailfold capillaroscopy, routine laboratory tests and autoantibodies. Conditions resembling Raynaud's that further need to be distinguished include acrocyanosis, a condition characterized by continuous cyanosis of the hands or feet that is aggravated by cold temperature, and erythromelalgia, a very rare condition, featuring paroxysmal burning pain with marked reddening of the legs, feet and less often the hands. In the latter case, attacks are triggered by warmth [5].

Distinction between primary and secondary Raynaud's phenomenon is of particular clinical importance, since patients with secondary Raynaud characterized by not mere vasospasm, but also fixed vascular defects and more severe ischemia, require further medical evaluation and potential treatment.

To accurately diagnose and differentiate Raynaud's phenomenon several methods have been proposed. Provocation of Raynaud through immersion of the hands in cold water may induce the phenomenon, but is not always reliable; it is considered a relatively sensitive diagnostic method in patients with the hand-vibration syndrome. Thermography, a method which has been for the assessment of the patient with Raynaud in specialist centres for over 25 yrs, employs an infrared camera to measure the temperature distribution of the skin by detecting its natural thermal radiation, thus giving an indirect record of micro- and macro-vascular flow, as the blood carries heat to the imaged area [33]. However, the technique has limitations, mainly regarding reproducibility of its results [34-36]. To improve the specificity of this technique and increase its potential in the differential diagnosis of secondary from primary Raynaud's, the evaluation of the "distal-dorsal difference" was proposed; this parameter was found to be specific (83%), but lacked sensitivity (69%) for the diagnosis of secondary Raynaud's phenomenon [37]. Other methodologies have been proposed for the classification of Raynaud's phenomenon, e.g. based on angiographic features [38].

The mainstay of screening techniques for the diagnosis of seconday Raynaud remains the in vivo nailfold capillaroscopy. Imaging with nailfold videocapillaroscopy (NVC) enables the early differentiation between primary and secondary Raynaud's phenomenon by identifying morphological patterns specific to various stages of systemic sclerosis ('early', 'active' and 'late' patterns) [39] and/ or other rheumatologic conditions; pathognomonic vascular capillaroscopic findings have been recently integrated as a criterion for the diagnosis of systemic sclerosis in the reformed EUSTAR/EULAR guidelines [40].

## NAILFOLD CAPILLAROSCOPY; THE TECHNIQUE AND ITS EVOLUTION

The technique of capillaroscopy has been applied since the 18$^{th}$ century, when Giovanni Rasori reported for the first time an association between conjuctival inflammation and the presence of an "inextrictable knot of capillary loops" by a magnifying glass [41]. Pathological findings in this first description were characterized as abnormally reddish. The observation of human periungual skin capillaries by Lombard in 1911 was next to follow [42]. The abnormalities characterizing the microvasculature in systemic sclerosis were analytically described for the time in 1925 by Brown and O' Leary. The identification of characteristic microvascular abnormalities raised a philosophical dispute to the theory of Raynaud, who beleieved Raynaud to be a defect in the innervation of small vessels, rather than an established structural abnormality. Since the 1930s capillaroscopy was temporarily neglected for a few decades, mainly due to the lack of practical capillaroscopic systems, only to be reinstituted later as a valuable aid in the diagnosis of connective tissue diseases and vascular acrosyndromes in general [43, 44].

The technique of capillaroscopy has evolved impressively throughout the centuries. Following the magnifying glass of Giovanni Rasori soon the technique was set (with the aid of an ophthalmoscope or a stereoscope) and pictures were recorded on camera [45]. Modern capillaroscopic devices comprise of a contact lens which transfers the nailfold capillary bed images through optic fibers to a computer system, where images can be stored, analyzed and compared. The undisputed advantage of the recent devices is flexibility, which allows examination to be performed in direct contact with the human body, and at the bedside [46]. The incorporation of a video system and software for digital image analysis allowed the evaluation of the function of the capillary bed, by determining capillary haemodynamics and exchanges besides the quantitative appraisal of microangiopathies. The insertion of fluorescent dyes and the subsequent performance of fluorescent video capillaroscopy further enhances the in vivo evaluation of the functional status of skin microcirculation by detecting nailfold capillary hemodynamics as well as transcapillary and interstitial diffusion of sodium fluorescein [47].

## Nailfold Capillaroscopy as a Screening Clinical Tool

As mentioned previously, Raynaud affects 2-22% of the general population. There is general agreement that every patient with Raynaud should undergo a capillaroscopic examination to characterize the present clinical and evolving profile [48]. Examination is performed at room temperature with the patient seated comfortably and relaxed, resting his hand on a firm tabloid. All fingers but the thumb are consecutively examined. In the healthy subject, the nailfold capillary bed shows a regular architecture, and capillaries appear with uniform shape, distribution and diameter, most of them showing a hairpin or U shaped structure. (Figure 1).

Capillaroscopic findings associated with Raynaud's phenomenon may vary, ranging from a normal pattern (idiopathic Raynaud) to abnormalities that show microvascular involvement, including microhemorrhages, irregularly enlarged loops, megacapillaries or giant loops, neoangiogenesis, architectural derangement, and loss of capillaries [49-52], Figure 2.

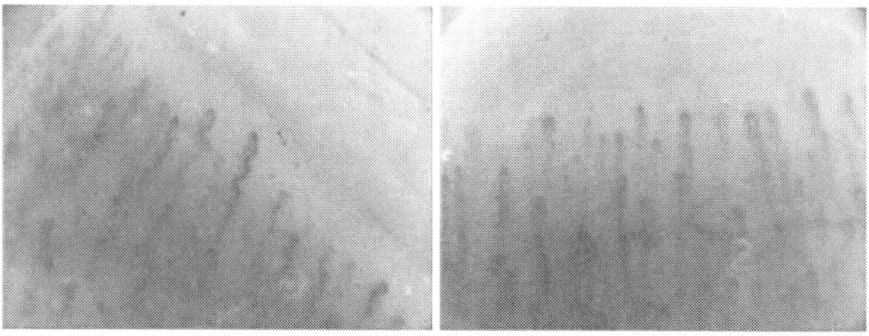

A B

Figure 1. A, B. Normal capillaroscopic pattern; regular architecture of the capillary bed, hairpin or U-shaped structure of the capillaries.

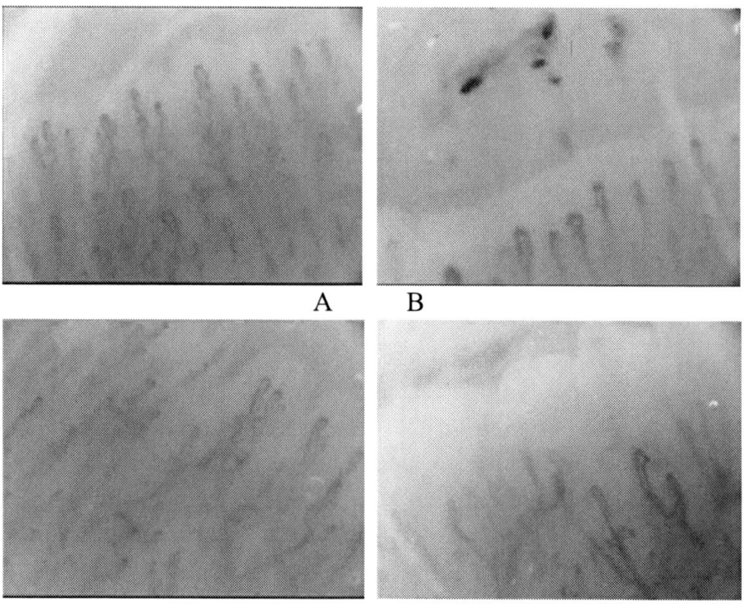


C D

Figure 2. A-D. Pathological capillaroscopic patterns; A. capillary tortuosity, B. enlargement of capillaries with hemorrhages, C. neovascularization and D. structural derrangement of the nailfold capillary bed.

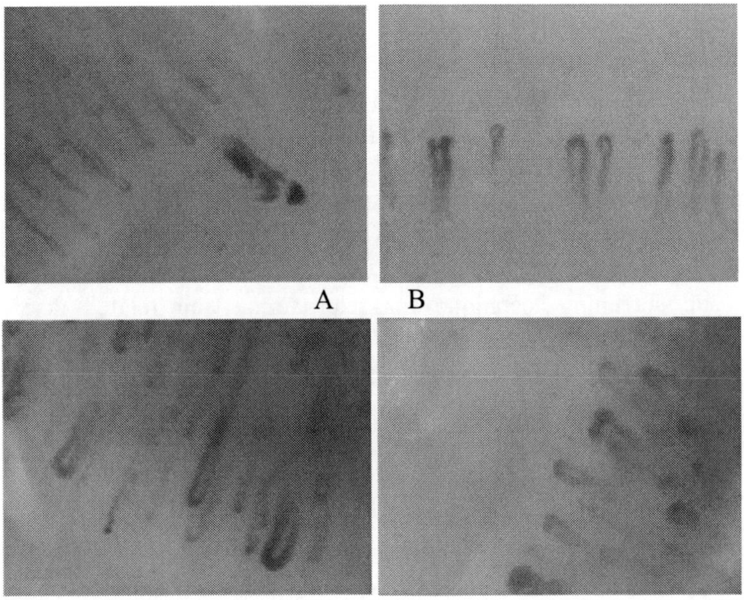
A B
C D

Figure 3. A-D. "Early" scleroderma pattern; A. microhemorrhages, B-D. enlargement of capillaries. A-D. relative preservation of capillary density.

In patients with Raynaud, and lack of other clinical manifestations, even isolated morphologic abnormalities such as a megacapillary or an irregularly enlarged loop should alert the physician to the possibility of an underlying scleroderma spectrum disorder (secondary Raynaud) [41]; approximately 15 to 20% of individuals with Raynaud's phenomenon who have microcirculatory alterations (assessed by capillaroscopy) and/or autoantibodies, and do not meet criteria at presentation, will develop a connective tissue disease within two years (not meeting criteria at baseline); [53].

The most characteristic and recognizable pathologic capillaroscopic pattern is that of the scleroderma spectrum disorder (including systemic sclerosis, dermatomyositis and mixed connective tissue disease); [54]. Three different patterns can be recognized in these patients. The "early" scleroderma pattern, usually accompanied by Raynaud's phenomenon as the sole clinical feature of the disease, is characterized by few enlarged/giant capillaries, few capillary haemorrhages, relatively well-preserved capillary distribution and no evident loss of capillaries (Figure 3A-D). In the "active" scleroderma pattern giant capillaries and associated capillary haemorrhages are frequently observed, with moderate loss of capillary density, mild disorganization of the capillary architecture and absent or mild ramified capillaries (Figure 4A-D). Finally, the advanced or "late" scleroderma capillaroscopic pattern is characterized by severe loss of capillaries resulting in extensive avascular areas. The capillary array is disorganized, ramified/bushy capillaries are commonly found, and giant capillaries or haemorrhages are few or absent. The scleroderma-type pattern can also be observed in the other scleroderma spectrum disorders (dermatomyositis and mixed connective tissue disease). Capillaroscopy is a very sensitive (>90%) and relatively specific (63.5%) diagnostic screening technique for scleroderma and related diseases; its negative predictive value reaches 96.7%, rendering capillaroscopy a valuable technique to rule out the presence of analogous disorders [55]. When corresponding capillaroscopic findings are added to the other scleroderma diagnostic criteria they increase the sensitivity of the diagnosis to up to 99% [56]. Capillary abnormalities can be observed in other rheumatic diseases, cannot however be characterized as pathognomonic in these conditions. Although findings are usually similar to healthy subjects (~50%), patients with systemic lupus erythematosus may exhibit elongated capillaries, increased tortuosity, a prominent subpapillary plexus and granular flow [57, 58].

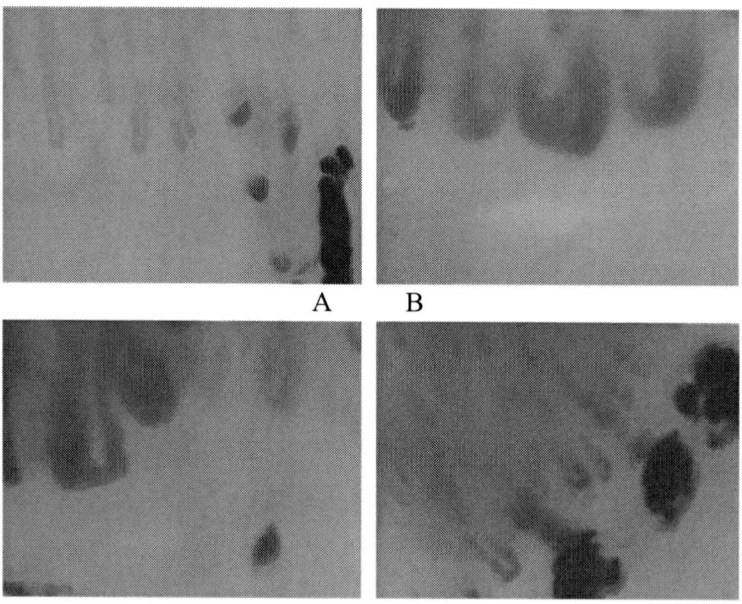

A B

C D

Figure 4. A-D. "Active" scleroderma pattern; frequent hemorrhages, "giant" capillaries and reduction of capillary density.

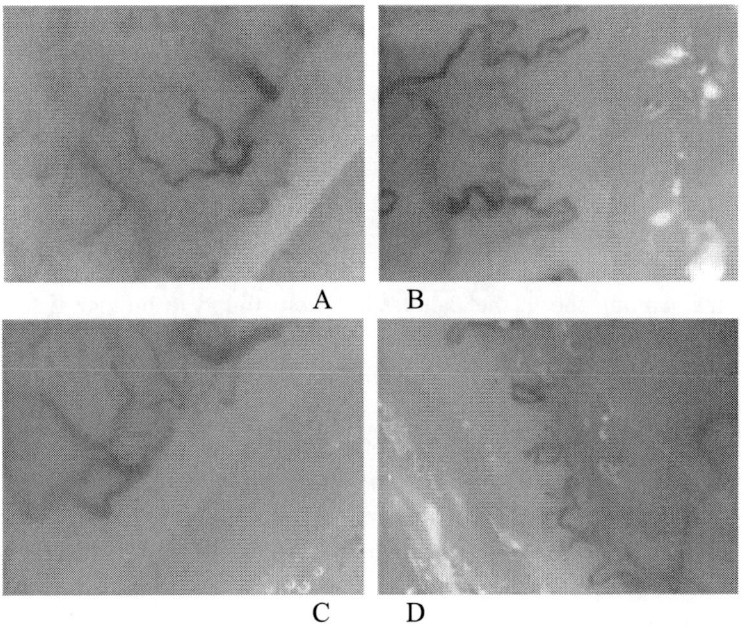


Figure 5. A-D. "Late" scleroderma pattern; severe reduction of capillary density, ramified capillaries.

Patients with Sjogren's syndrome may exhibit non-specific abnormalities (dilated, abnormal, and meandering capillaries, capillary hemorrhages and venous plexus visibility); [59]. In patients with antiphospholipid syndrome, capillary tortuosity was observed more frequently than in healthy controls [60]. Moreover, capillary diameter was found to be significantly smaller than in controls, although no difference was found in capillary density or blood flow velocity [61]. Symmetrical microhemorrhages at nailfold capillaroscopic analysis may be observed, and these alterations were found to be particularly significant in patients with both IgG and IgM anticardiolipin antibodies and a history of thrombotic manifestations [62-65].

## Nailfold Capillaroscopy as a Clinical Prognostic Tool

To assess the potential of nailfold capillaroscopy to predict clinical manifestations of rheumatic diseases, 3029 patients with primary Raynaud were reassessed every 6 months for a mean total period of 4.8 years [66].

Pathological capillaroscopic findings were recorded in all patients in the absence of clinical and serological signs of connective tissue diseases. In patients who progressed to develop connective tissue diseases, retrospective analysis of the capillaroscopic pattern 6 months prior to the manifestation of the symptomatology revealed statistically significant association of pathological capillaroscopic findings with progression to a disease of the scleroderma spectrum. The PRINCE study assessed the prognostic value of each isolated pathological capillaroscopic finding in patients with isopated Raynaud. Among those, the factors that were found to be significant in the prediction of transition to a disease of the scleroderma spectrum disorder was the presence of giant loops, microhemorrhages, and the number of capillaries [52].

Besides prediction of the development of connective tissue diseases in otherwise healthy individuals with isolated Raynaud's phenomenon, capillaroscopical assessment appears to provide an additional clinical evaluation tool to predict disease subset (manifestations) and severity in the follow-up of patients with established diagnosis. In a study involving 103 Italian patients with limited and diffuse scleroderma it was found that severity of skin, lung, heart and peripheral vascular involvement progressively increased across nailfold videocapillaroscopic patterns, from early to late pattern [67]. In the same study, patients exhibiting late pattern showed an increased risk to have active disease, to develop digital ulcers and moderate to severe skin, heart, and lung involvement. This may indicate a putative role of capillaroscopy as a biomarker. Similar observations in pilot prospective studies qualify capillaroscopy as a potential biomarker in analogous patients [68]. Interestingly, specific, but not all, oxidative stress parameters appear to relate with advanced microvascular damage and corresponding capillaroscopic images in scleroderma patients [69].

Recently, a new clinical marker, the capillaroscopic skin ulcer risk index (CSURI), was developed, in order to predict the onset of new digital ulcers in scleroderma patients based on capillarospic findings [70]. For the estimation of CSURI the total number of analyzed capillaries in the distal row (N), the number of megacapillaries (M), the M:N ratio, the maximum diameter of megacapillaries (D), and the presence or absence of tortuosities and microhemorrhages are inserted in the equation (M:NxD): N, simplified to $DxM:N^2$. Interestingly, the appearance of new ulcers did not correlate with microhemorrhages, capillary tortuosities, autoantibodies, cutaneous scleroderma subsets, and scleroderma and Raynaud's phenomenon durations. Patients with new digital ulcers showed a mean ±SD CSURI of 13.286

±16.132, versus 3.185 ±9.386 in patients without new ischemic lesions. With a cutoff value of 2.94, the positive predictive value of CSURI was 73.33%. Previous discordant results, failing to associate capillaroscopic results with prognostic information and visceral involvement in patients with scleroderma [50, 71] could possibly be attributed to differences in patient selection, the quantification methods of clinical and capillaroscopic alterations, and/or technical limitations; newly developed computer-based technology showed a low interoperator variability, allowing objective semi-quantitative assessments [72].

## Nailfold Capillaroscopy as a Treatment Response Predictor

The issue was bound to come up; would treatment reverse pathological nailfold capillaroscopy images? To address it, scleroderma patients were evaluated at baseline, and assigned to receive a non-selective endothelin antagonist, which may not promote the healing of existing digital ulcers, but has been proven to prevent the development of new ulcers [73-75]. Accutely after initiation of treatment, and at the end of the study (after 24 weeks of treatment), markers of microvascular structure and function, such as Laser Doppler imaging, systolic finger pressures and nailfold capillaroscopic imaging were reassessed [76].

In this study, and for the specific time-frame of treatment, none of the parameters measured was significantly different, and there was no evidence of any linear trends. Potential caveats of the study were the lack of a control/ placebo arm, the relative short duration of the study and the lack of patients with ealier stage of the disease.

An anecdotal report exists in the literature indicating a direct and imminent effect of intravenous iloprost (a prostacyclin analogue) administration on microvascular morphology in a patient with acute Raynaud [77]. Prostacyclin analogues have proved to be effective agents in the healing process of existing digital ulcers [78] and are believed to have vascular remodelling properties [79]. A pilot study was designed to investigate whether intravenous prostanoids, which are currently the mainstay of treatment for severe SSc-related digital ischemia, may be associated with structural changes in the digital microvasculature as quantified by nailfold videocapillaroscopy. Nine patients were included in the study with the indication of progressive skin thickening and one with concomitant forearm ulceration. Nailfold capillary assessment was performed at baseline, day 3 and day 5 of treatment, and 12 months post iloprost. While there was a trend for capillary density to increase immediately following iloprost , this was not sustained at 12 months. There was a trend toward a decrease in apical width 12 months post-iloprost. As technology improves, biochemical and serological markers are becoming identified and their pathophysiological role deciphered, and new targeted therapies are being developed, nailfold capillaroscopy will undoubtedly prove to be a valuable aid in the screening, evaluation and follow-up of diseases whose pathophysiology relies on microvasculature damage.

## References


[1] Bakst R, Merola JF, Franks AG Jr, Sanchez M. Raynaud's phenomenon: pathogenesis and management. *J. Am. Acad. Dermatol.* 2008 Oct; 59(4): 633-53. Epub 2008 Jul 24.

[2] Chikura B, Moore TL, Manning JB, Vail A, Herrick AL. Sparing of the thumb in Raynaud's phenomenon. *Rheumatology* (Oxford). 2008 Feb;47(2):219-21.

[3] Goldman W, Seltzer R, Reuman P. Association between treatment with central nervous system stimulants and Raynaud's syndrome in children: a retrospective case-control study of rheumatology patients. *Arthritis Rheum.* 2008 Feb;58(2):563-6.

[4] Fonseca C, Abraham D, Ponticos M. Neuronal regulators and vascular dysfunction in Raynaud's phenomenon and systemic sclerosis. *Curr. Vasc. Pharmacol.* 2009 Jan;7(1):34-9.

[5] Heidrich H. Functional vascular diseases: Raynaud's syndrome, acrocyanosis and erythromelalgia. *VASA* 2010;39:33-41.

[6] Bollinger A, Schlumpf M. Finger blood flow in healthy subjects of different age and sex and in patients with primary Raynaud's disease. *Acta Chir. Scand. Suppl.* 1976; 465: 42-47.

[7] Cooke JP, Creager MA, Osmundson PJ, Shepherd JT. Sex differences in control of cutaneous blood flow. Circulation 1990; 82: 1607-1615.

[8] Freedman RR, Girgis R. Effects of menstrual cycle and race on peripheral vascular alpha-adrenergic responsiveness. *Hypertension* 2000; 35: 795-799.

[9] Thompson CS, Kenney WL. Altered neurotransmitter control of reflex vasoconstriction in aged human skin. *J. Physiol.* 2004;558:697–704.

[10] Holowatz LA, Thompson-Torgerson C, and Kenney LW. Aging and the control of human skin blood flow. *Front Biosci.* 2010 January 1; 15: 718–739.

[11] Maricq HR, Carpentier PH, Weinrich MC, Keil JE, Franco A, Drouet P, et al. Geographic variation in the prevalence of Raynaud's phenomenon: Charleston, SC, USA, vs Tarentaise, Savoie, France. *J. Rheumatol.* 1993; 20:70–6.

[12] Cherkas LF, Williams FM, Carter L, Howell K, Black CM, Spector TD, et al. Heritability of Raynaud's phenomenon and vascular responsiveness to cold: a study of adult female twins. *Arthritis Rheum.* 2007 Apr 15; 57(3):524-8.

[13] Suter LG, Murabito JM, Felson DT, Fraenkel L. The incidence and natural history of Raynaud's phenomenon in the community. *Arthritis Rheum.* 2005 Apr;52(4):1259-63.

[14] Gelber AC, Wigley FM, Stallings RY, Bone LR, Barker AV, Baylor I, et al. Symptoms of Raynaud's phenomenon in an inner-city African-American community: prevalence and selfreported cardiovascular comorbidity. *J. Clin. Epidemiol.* 1999;52: 441–6.

[15] O'Keeffe ST, Tsapatsaris NP, Beetham WP Jr. Color chart assisted diagnosis of Raynaud's phenomenon in an unselected hospital employee population. *J. Rheumatol.* 1992;19:1415–7.

[16] Weinrich MC, Maricq HR, Keil JE, McGregor AR, Diat F. Prevalence of Raynaud phenomenon in the adult population of South Carolina. *J. Clin. Epidemiol.* 1990;43:1343- 9.

[17] Thériault G, De Guire L, Gingras S, Laroche G. Raynaud's phenomenon in forestry workers in Quebec. *Can. Med. Assoc. J.* 1982 Jun 15;126(12): 1404-8.

[18] Palmer K, Griffin M., Syddall H., Pannett B., Cooper C., Coggon D. Prevalence of Raynaud's phenomenon in Great Britain and its relation to hand transmitted vibration: a national postal survey. *Occup. Environ. Med.* 2000 July; 57(7): 448–452.

[19] Roquelaure Y, Ha C, Le Manac'h AP, Bodin J, Bodere A, Bosseau C, et al. Risk factors for Raynaud's phenomenon in the workforce. *Arthritis Care Res.* (Hoboken). 2012 Jun;64(6):898-904. doi: 10.1002/acr.21615. Epub 2012 Jan 13.

[20] Keil JE, Maricq HR, Weinrich MC, McGregor AR, Diat F. Demographic, social and clinical correlates of Raynaud phenomenon. *Int. J. Epidemiol.* 1991 Mar;20(1):221-4.

[21] Cherniack M, Clive J, Seidner A. Vibration exposure, smoking, and vascular dysfunction. *Occup. Environ. Med.* 2000;57:341–7.
[22] Harrison BJ, Silman AJ, Hider SL, Herrick AL. Cigarette smoking: a significant risk factor for digital vascular diseases in patients with systemic sclerosis. *Arthritis Rheum.* 2002;46:3312–6.
[23] Palesch YY, Valter I, Carpentier PH, Maricq HR. Association between cigarette and alcohol consumption and Raynaud's phenomenon. *J. Clin. Epidemiol.* 1999 Apr;52(4):321-8.
[24] Herrick AL. Pathogenesis of Raynaud's phenomenon. *Rheumatology* (Oxford). 2005 May;44(5):587-96. Epub 2005 Mar 1.
[25] Al-Allaf A-W, Belch JJF. Raynaud's phenomenon. In: Hochberg MC, Silman AJ, Smolen JS et al., eds. *Rheumatology*, 3rd edn. Elsevier, Edinburgh, 2003;1507–1512.
[26] Block JA, Sequeira W. Raynaud's phenomenon. *Lancet* 2001; 357: 2042–8.
[27] Hirschl M, Hirschl K, Lenz M, Katzenschlager R, Hutter HP, Kundi M. Transition from primary Raynaud's phenomenon to secondary Raynaud's phenomenon identified by diagnosis of an associated disease: results of ten years of prospective surveillance. *Arthritis Rheum.* 2006 Jun;54(6): 1974-81.
[28] Hirschl M, Kundi M. Initial prevalence and incidence of secondary Raynaud's phenomenon in patients with Raynaud's symptomatology. *J. Rheumatol.* 1996 Feb;23(2):302-9.
[29] LeRoy EC, Medsger TA Jr. Raynaud's phenomenon: a proposal for classification. *Clin. Exp. Rheumatol.* 1992 Sep-Oct;10(5):485-8.
[30] Jones GT, Herrick AL, Woodham SE, Baildam EM, Macfarlane GJ, Silman AJ. Occurrence of Raynaud's phenomenon in children ages 12-15 years: prevalence and association with other common symptoms. *Arthritis Rheum.* 2003 Dec;48(12):3518-21.
[31] Zeni S, Ingegnoli F. [Raynaud's phenomenon]. *Reumatismo.* 2004 Apr-Jun;56(2):77-81.
[32] Gayraud M. Raynaud's phenomenon. *Joint Bone Spine.* 2007 Jan;74(1): e1-8. Epub 2006 Dec 4.
[33] Jones BF. A reappraisal of the use of infrared thermal image analysis in medicine. *IEEE Transactions Med. Imaging* 1998;17:1019-27.
[34] Chucker F, Fowler RC, Motomiya T, Singh B, Hurley W. Induced temperature transients in Raynaud's disease measured by thermography. A preliminary report. *Angiology* 1971;22:580-93.

[35] Chucker FD, Fowler RC, Hurley CW. Photoplethysmometry and thermography in Raynaud's disorders. A preliminary report. *Angiology* 1973;24:612-8.

[36] Herrick A, el-Hadidy K, Marsh D, Jayson M. Abnormal thermoregulatory responses in patients with reflex sympathetic dystrophy syndrome. *J. Rheumatol.* 1994;21:1319-24.

[37] Anderson ME, Moore TL, Lunt M, Herrick AL. The 'distal-dorsal difference': a thermographic parameter by which to differentiate between primary and secondary Raynaud's phenomenon. *Rheumatology* (Oxford). 2007 Mar;46(3):533-8. Epub 2006 Oct 2.

[38] Kim YH, Ng SW, Seo HS, Chang Ahn H. Classification of Raynaud's disease based on angiographic features. *J. Plast. Reconstr. Aesthet. Surg.* 2011 Nov;64(11):1503-11. Epub 2011 Jun 24.

[39] Cutolo M, Sulli A, Smith V. Assessing microvascular changes in systemic sclerosis diagnosis and management. *Nat. Rev. Rheumatol.* 2010 Oct;6(10):578-87. Epub 2010 Aug 10.

[40] Avouac J, Fransen J, Walker UA, Riccieri V, Smith V, Muller C, et al; EUSTAR Group. Preliminary criteria for the very early diagnosis of systemic sclerosis: results of a Delphi Consensus Study from EULAR Scleroderma Trials and Research Group. *Ann. Rheum. Dis.* 2011 Mar; 70(3): 476-81. Epub 2010 Nov 15.

[41] Cutolo M, Grassi W, Matucci Cerinic M. Raynaud's phenomenon and the role of capillaroscopy. *Arthritis Rheum.* 2003;48:3023–30.

[42] Lombard WP. The blood pressure in the arterioles, capillaries, and small veins of the human skin. *Am. J. Physiol.* 1911;29:355–62.

[43] Ross JB. Nail fold capillaroscopy--a useful aid in the diagnosis of collagen vascular diseases. *J. Invest. Dermatol.* 1966 Oct;47(4):282-5.

[44] Merlen JF, Hiltenbrand C, Coget J. [Nail-bed and ocular conjunctiva capillaroscopy in the diagnosis of vascular acrosyndromes]. *Ann. Cardiol. Angeiol.* (Paris). 1969 Apr-Jun;18(2):161-5.

[45] Weiss W. Demonstration von Hautkapillarveraenderungen bei akuter Nephritis. *Med. Bl Landerver* 1916;LXXXVI:383.

[46] Carpentier PH. New techniques for clinical assessment of the peripheral microcirculation. *Drugs.* 1999;59 Spec No:17-22.

[47] Bollinger A, Ja¨ger K, Roten A, Timeus C, Mahler F. Diffusion, pericapillary distribution and clearance of Na-fluorescein in the human nailfold. *Pflugers Arch.* 1979;382:137–43.

[48] De Angelis R, Grassi W, Cutolo M. A growing need for capillaroscopy in rheumatology. *Arthritis Rheum.* 2009 Mar 15;61(3):405-10.

[49] Maricq HR, LeRoy EC. Patterns of finger capillary abnormalities in connective tissue disease by "wide-field" microscopy. *Arthritis Rheum.* 1973; 16:619–28.

[50] Lovy M, MacCarter D, Steigerwald JC. Relationship between nailfold capillary abnormalities and organ involvement in systemic sclerosis. *Arthritis Rheum.* 1985;28:496–501.

[51] Houtman PM, Kallenberg CG, Fidler V, Wouda AA. Diagnostic significance of nailfold capillary patterns in patients with Raynaud's phenomenon. *J. Rheumatol.* 1986;13:556–63.

[52] Ingegnoli F, Boracchi P, Gualtierotti R, Lubatti C, Meani L, Zahalkova L, et al. Prognostic model based on nailfold capillaroscopy for identifying Raynaud's phenomenon patients at high risk for the development of a scleroderma spectrum disorder: PRINCE (Prognostic Index for Nailfold Capillaroscopic Examination). *Arthritis Rheum.* 2008; 58:2174–82.

[53] Zuffery P, Depairon M, Chamot AM, Monti M. Prognostic significance of nailfold capillary microscopy in patients with Raynaud's phenomenon and scleroderma-pattern abnormalities: a six-year follow-up study. *Clin. Rheumatol.* 1992;11:536-541.

[54] Maricq HR, Harper FE, Khan MM, Tan EM, LeRoy EC. Microvascular abnormalities as possible predictors of disease subsets in Raynaud's phenomenon and early connective tissue disease. *Clin. Exp. Rheumatol.* 1983;1:195–205.

[55] Blockmans D, Beyens G, Verhaeghe R. Predictive value of nailfold capillaroscopy in the diagnosis of connective tissue diseases. *Clin. Rheumatol.* 1996 Mar;15(2):148-53.

[56] Hudson M, Taillefer S, Steele R, Dunne J, Johnson SR, Jones N, et al. Improving the sensitivity of the American College of Rheumatology classification criteria for systemic sclerosis. *Clin. Exp. Rheumatol.* 2007 Sep-Oct;25(5):754-7.

[57] Lambova SN, Müller-Ladner U. Capillaroscopic pattern in systemic lupus erythematosus and undifferentiated connective tissue disease: What we still have to learn? *Rheumatol. Int.* 2012 Apr 24. [Epub ahead of print].

[58] Pavlov-Dolijanovic S, Damjanov NS, Vujasinovic Stupar NZ, Marcetic DR, Sefik-Bukilica MN, Petrovic RR. Is there a difference in systemic lupus erythematosus with and without Raynaud's phenomenon? *Rheumatol. Int.* 2012 May 22. [Epub ahead of print].

[59] Capobianco KG, Xavier RM, Bredemeier M, Restelli VG, Brenol JC. Nailfold capillaroscopic findings in primary Sjögren's syndrome: clinical and serological correlations. *Clin. Exp. Rheumatol.* 2005 Nov-Dec; 23(6): 789-94.

[60] Vaz JL, Dancour MA, Bottino DA, Bouskela E. Nailfold videocapillaroscopy in primary antiphospholipid syndrome (PAPS). *Rheumatology* (Oxford) 2004; 43:1025-1027.

[61] Cortes S, Cutolo M. Capillarosecopic patterns in rheumatic diseases. *Acta Reumatol. Port.* 2007 Jan-Mar;32(1):29-36.

[62] Sulli A, Pizzorni C, Cutolo M. Nailfold videocapillaroscopy abnormalities in patients with antiphospholipid antibodies. *J. Rheumatol.* 2000;27:1574-1576.

[63] Pyrpasopoulou A, Triantafyllou A, Anyfanti P, Douma S, Aslanidis S. Capillaroscopy as a screening test for clinical antiphospholipid syndrome. *Eur. J. Intern. Med.* 2011 Dec;22(6):e158-9. Epub 2011 Aug 11. No abstract available.

[64] Aslanidis S, Pyrpasopoulou A, Doumas M, Triantafyllou A, Chatzimichailidou S, Zamboulis C. Association of capillaroscopic microhaemorrhages with clinical and immunological antiphospholipid syndrome. *Clin. Exp. Rheumatol.* 2011 Mar-Apr;29(2):307-9. Epub 2011 Apr 19.

[65] Candela M, Pansoni A, De Carolis ST, Pomponio G, Corvetta A, Gabrielli A, et al. [Nailfold capillary microscopy in patients with antiphospholipid syndrome]. *Recenti. Prog. Med.* 1998 Sep;89(9):444-9.

[66] Pavlov-Dolijanovic S, Damjanov NS, Stojanovic RM, Vujasinovic Stupar NZ, Stanisavljevic DM. Scleroderma pattern of nailfold capillary changes as predictive value for the development of a connective tissue disease: a follow-up study of 3,029 patients with primary Raynaud's phenomenon. *Rheumatol. Int.* 2012 Oct;32(10):3039-45. Epub 2011 Sep 8.

[67] Caramaschi P, Canestrini S, Martinelli N, Volpe A, Pieropan S, Ferrari M, et al. Scleroderma patients nailfold videocapillaroscopic patterns are associated with disease subset and disease severity. *Rheumatology* (Oxford). 2007 Oct;46(10):1566-9. Epub 2007 Aug 10.

[68] Smith V, Decuman S, Sulli A, Bonroy C, Piettte Y, Deschepper E, et al. Do worsening scleroderma capillaroscopic patterns predict future severe organ involvement? a pilot study. *Ann. Rheum. Dis.* 2012 Oct;71(10): 1636-9. doi: 10.1136/annrheumdis-2011-200780. Epub 2012 Mar 8.

[69] Riccieri V, Spadaro A, Fuksa L, Firuzi O, Saso L, Valesini G. Specific oxidative stress parameters differently correlate with nailfold capillaroscopy changes and organ involvement in systemic sclerosis. *Clin. Rheumatol.* 2008 Feb;27(2):225-30. Epub 2007 Oct 27.

[70] Sebastiani M, Manfredi A, Colaci M, D'amico R, Malagoli V, Giuggioli D, et al. Capillaroscopic skin ulcer risk index: a new prognostic tool for digital skin ulcer development in systemic sclerosis patients. *Arthritis Rheum.* 2009 May 15;61(5):688-94.

[71] Statham BN, Rowell NR. Quantification of the nail fold capillary abnormalities in systemic sclerosis and Raynaud's syndrome. *Acta Derm. Venereol.* 1986;66:139–43.

[72] Scheja A, Akesson A, Niewierowicz I, Wallin L, Wildt M, Wollheim FA. Computer based quantitative analysis of capillary abnormalities in systemic sclerosis and its relation to plasma concentration of von Willebrand factor. *Ann. Rheum. Dis.* 1996;55:52–6.

[73] Roman Ivorra JA, Simeon CP, Alegre Sancho JJ, Egurbide MV, Castillo MJ, Lloria X, et al. Bosentan in clinical practice for treating digital and other ischemic ulcers in Spanish patients with systemic sclerosis: IBER-DU cohort study *J. Rheumatol.* 2011 Aug;38(8):1631-5. Epub 2011 Jun 1.

[74] Matucci-Cerinic M, Denton CP, Furst DE, Mayes MD, Hsu VM, Carpentier P, et al. Bosentan treatment of digital ulcers related to systemic sclerosis: results from the RAPIDS-2 randomised, double-blind, placebo-controlled trial. *Ann. Rheum. Dis.* 2011 Jan;70(1):32-8. Epub 2010 Aug 30.

[75] Steen V, Denton CP, Pope JE, Matucci-Cerinic M. Digital ulcers: overt vascular disease in systemic sclerosis. *Rheumatology* (Oxford). 2009 Jun;48 Suppl 3:iii19-24.

[76] Moore TL, Vail A, Herrick AL. Assessment of digital vascular structure and function in response to bosentan in patients with systemic sclerosis-related Raynaud's phenomenon. *Rheumatology* (Oxford). 2007 Feb; 46(2): 363-4. Epub 2006 Nov 20.

[77] Pyrpasopoulou A, Aslanidis S. Clinical images: iloprost-induced vascular remodeling. *Arthritis Rheum.* 2007 Jul;56(7):2243. No abstract available.

[78] Kawald A, Burmester GR, Huscher D, Sunderkötter C, Riemekasten G. Low versus high-dose iloprost therapy over 21 days in patients with secondary Raynaud's phenomenon and systemic sclerosis: a randomized, open, single-center study. *J. Rheumatol.* 2008 Sep;35(9):1830-7. Epub 2008 Jul 15.

[79] Fishman AP. Pulmonary hypertension — beyond vasodilator therapy. *N. Engl. J. Med.* 1998;338:321–2.

In: Screening Tests
Editor: Marguerite Gauthier

ISBN: 978-1-62417-963-1
© 2013 Nova Science Publishers, Inc.

*Chapter 4*

# THE FACTORIAL STRUCTURE OF THE SHORT FORM PROFILE OF MOODS SCALE

***Julie Aitken Schermer[1,*] and David R. Cann[2]***

[1]Management and Organizational Studies, Social Sciences
The University of Western Ontario, London, Ontario, Canada
[2]Department of Psychology, Mount Royal University
Calgary, Alberta, Canada

## ABSTRACT

The factorial structure of the short form Profile of Moods Scale (POMS; McNair, Lorr, and Droppleman, 1992) was examined based on responses to the scale by 290 adults (122 men and 168 women). The short form POMS is a 30-item scale designed to assess six dimensions of mood: Vigor, Tension, Fatigue, Depression, Confusion, and Anger. The short form of the POMS was derived from the longer 65-item scale which was developed using factor analytic techniques, although this statistical method was not used in the generation of the short form of the scale. Following an analysis of the factorial structure of the short form items, five of the six scales were found to fit the proposed pattern; the exception was for the items measuring Confusion.

* E-mail: jharris@uwo.ca.

# INTRODUCTION

Research focused on understanding mood and emotion has been popular the past few decades. For example, Watson and Clark (1997) reported 1,857 articles published between 1994 and 1997 based on a PsycLIT database search using the keywords "mood" or "emotion". A recent search of the PsycInfo database using the same keywords revealed over 20,500 published articles for the years 2000 to 2012. As Watson and Clark (1997) noted, such growth in this research domain necessitates reliable and valid measures in which to assess the underlying constructs. One commonly used measure, in relation to mood assessment, is the Profile of Mood States questionnaire (POMS: McNair, Lorr, and Droppleman, 1971; 1992). McNair, Heuchert, and Shilony (2003) reported that the POMS had been used in over 2,900 research studies; thus indicating the popularity of this measure in mood-related research.

The POMS has seen wide-spread use across a multitude of research domains and has been translated into numerous languages. For example, Bourgeois LeUnes, and Meyers (2010) indicate that the POMS has been translated into Chinese, Czech, French, German, Italian, Japanese, Korean, and Spanish. In addition, Aroian, Kulwicki, Kaskiri, Templin, and Wells (2007) report the psychometric properties of an Arabic version. The POMS has also been used to assess mood in a variety of clinical and non-clinical populations including: college students (e.g., Boyle, 1987,1988; Miller and Edginton, 1984) athletes (for a review see Berger and Motl, 2000; LeUnes, 2000; LeUnes and Burger, 1998); geriatric populations (e.g., Gibson, 1997; Kaye, Lawton, Gitlin, Kleban, Windsor, and Kaye, 1988); bone marrow transplant survivors (e.g., Curran, Andrykowski, and Studts, 1995); myocardial infarction patients (e.g., Fink, Eckhardt, Fennessy, Jones, Kruse, VanderZwan, Ryan, and Zerwic, 2010); postmenopausal women (e.g., Wyrwich and Yu, 2011); HIV patients (e.g., Patterson, Young, Woods, Vigil, Grant, Atkinson, et al., 2006); alcoholic patients (e.g., McMahon and Davidson, 1986); pregnant and postpartum women (e.g., Dipietro, Costigan, and Sipsma, 2008; Tunis, Golbus, Copeland, Fine, Rosinsky, and Seely, 1990); psychiatric populations (e.g., Jacobson, Weiss, Steinbook, Brauzer, and Goldstein, 1978; Norcross, Guadagnoli, and Prochaska, 1984); depression in medical residents (e.g., Hainer and Palesch, 1998); prison inmates (e.g., Reddon, Marceau, and Holden, 1985); and patients with various types of cancer (e.g., Baker, Denniston, Zabora, Polland, and Dudley, 2002; DiLorenzo, Bovbjerg, Montgomery, Valdimarsdottir, and Jacobsen, 1999; Guadagnoli and Mor, 1989; Meek, Nail, Barsevick, Schwartz, Stephen, Whitmer, Beck, Jones, and

Walker, 2000). Based on the examples cited, it is clear that the POMS is a popular mood measurement instrument and as Bourgeois et al. (2010) noted, "it can be safely stated, based on the wide use of the POMS, that it demonstrates user acceptance, a critical psychometric quality" (p. 356).

Various versions of the POMS have been employed in research and clinical settings. The original long-form POMS (McNair et al., 1992) consists of 65 adjectives. When the POMS was created, McNair et al. (1992) describe six studies in which the factorial structure of the scale was assessed. In these studies, between five and seven factors were reported and McNair et al. (1992) report that across these studies, six factors consistently appear. The six consistent factors or subscales are: tension-anxiety, depression-dejection, anger-hostility, vigor-activity, fatigue-inertia, and confusion-bewilderment. Bourgeois et al. (2010) reported that the seven item *Friendliness* factor is not psychometrically sound and typically not scored if included on the scale, thus leaving the long-form POMS with 58 scored items (see also Norcross et al., 1984).

A number of authors (e.g., Baker et al., 2002; DiLorenzo et al., 1999; Shacham, 1983) have suggested that the use of the long form POMS can be problematic at times. Specifically, the long form can be taxing on severely ill individuals due to the length of time it can take for completion. Length of the scale may also be an issue in research settings (both clinical and non-clinical) in which batteries of assessment instruments are being administered. In reaction to these issues, a number of researchers have created various shortened versions of the POMS. The short form versions of the POMS that have been developed contain between six and 40 items (e.g., Dean, Whelan and Meyers, 1990 as cited in Bourgeois et al., 2010; Grove and Prapavessis, 1992; Shacham, 1983; Terry, Keohane, and Lane, 1996) with the most popular of these being Shacham's (1983) version. In what follows, a review of the research focused on the psychometric properties of Shachan's (1983) short form version of the POMS will be outlined and then discussion will focus on another short form version of the POMS, developed by McNair et al. (1992), the authors of the original long form version of the POMS. An exploratory factor analysis on this latter short form version of the POMS will then be presented.

Regardless of whether the long form or a short form version of the POMS is employed, individuals respond to the degree to which each adjective describes how the individual has felt in the past week. Responses are given by participants using a 0 ("Not at all") to 4 ("Extremely") response scale. Scores for each of the six factors or mood states are calculated by summing the responses for each of the items on the respective subscales. A composite seventh score representing Total Mood Disturbance (TMD) can be calculated by summing the scores on five of the subscales and subtracting from the positively scored vigor-activity subscale (Baker at al., 2002). According to McNair et al. (1971, 1992) the POMS can be completed by healthy individuals in five to seven minutes though it can take considerably longer to complete (e.g., 15 to 20 minutes) by severely ill individuals, such as cancer patients (Shacham, 1983) or older individuals (Berger and Motl, 2000). Also of note is the influence of time of day when completing the POMS. For example, Hill and Hill (1991) indicate that the TMD score was significantly greater when the POMS was completed in the morning (8:30am) than when it was completed in the afternoon (4:15pm). Further, of the six subscales scores, two (*Tension* and *Depression*) were significantly greater in the morning than the afternoon. Although there were no other significant differences, the general trend across the other subscales was higher scores in the morning than in the afternoon with the exception of the *Vigor* subscale in which scores were numerically greater in the afternoon than the morning. In general, this would seem to indicate that circadian rhythms can, to some degree, influence scores on the POMS.

The initial attempt to construct a short form version of the POMS was reported by Shacham (1983) in order to assist in ease of administration for clinical patients in severe pain. To create this short form version, Shacham (1983) administered the long form POMS to a group of cancer patients ($n$ = 83) and then based on the internal consistency of the items and the face validity of the items reduced the 65 item version to a shorter 37 item version. Shacham (1983) reported that the 37 remaining items on the six subscales were: Depression = *unhappy, sad, blue, hopeless, discouraged, miserable, helpless* and *worthless*; Vigor = *lively, active, energetic, cheerful, full of pep,* and *vigorous*; Confusion = *confused, unable to concentrate, bewildered, forgetful,* and *uncertain about things*; Tension = *tense, on edge, uneasy, restless, nervous,* and *anxious*; Anger = *angry, peeved, grouchy, annoyed, resentful, bitter,* and *furious*; Fatigue = *worn-out, fatigued, exhausted, weary,* and *bushed*. Good to excellent internal reliability, based on coefficient alpha, was reported for each of the subscales (Depression = .91, Vigor = .87, Confusion = .82, Tension = .80, Anger = .89, and Fatigue = .87) and each of the short form subscales exhibited strong correlations (all $r$'s equal to or above .95) with the long form subscales (Depression = .97, Vigor = .97, Confusion = .96, Tension = .95, Anger = .97, and Fatigue = .98). Based on these findings, Shacham (1983) concluded that the POMS can be shortened from the original 65 items while maintaining the internal consistency of the instrument without losing information and would be a suitable alternative when time or patient limitations are of concern to the researcher or clinician.

Since Shacham's (1983) short form POMS was developed, the scale has been used quite extensively especially with medical populations (for a brief review see Curran et al., 1995). However, as Curran et al. (1995) note, based on the limited sample used by Shacham (1983), and that no psychometric properties were reported in much of the research using the short form version, further investigations of the psychometric properties of the short form version were warranted. As such, Curran et al. (1995) administered the long form POMS to 600 individuals in which one sample consisted of healthy adults ($n$ = 76) and five different samples of medical patients (e.g., breast cancer patients, $n$ = 46; renal transplant survivors, $n$ = 68; benign breast disease patients, $n$ = 115; bone marrow transplant survivors, $n$ = 210; and bone marrow transplant candidates, $n$ = 85). By using the long form POMS, Curran et al. (1995) were able to create the short form POMS subscales using the items identified by Shacham (1983) and compared them to the long form POMS subscales (see Curran et al. for an explanation of how they calculated reliability-corrected correlations because of the potential for spuriously high correlations given that there was overlap among items on the short form version and long form version). Curran et al. (1995) reported adequate to excellent coefficient alpha's (a test of the internal consistency of the scale which represents the average of all possible split-half correlations) ranging from .76 (Confusion subscale in the healthy adult sample) to .95 (Depression subscale in the healthy adult sample). Overall, they calculated 36 coefficient alpha's (six samples by six subscales) resulting in two values slightly below .80 and 24 values above .90. In general, Curran et al.'s (1995) results, using much larger and more diverse samples, converge with those of Shacham's (1983). Curran et al. (1995) conclude that Shacham's (1983) short form version of the POMS is an excellent alternative to the long form POMS and that the internal consistency of some of the subscales on the short form may be better than their counterparts on the long form POMS.

DiLorenzo et al. (1999) also found similar psychometric properties between the long form POMS and the Shacham's (1983) short form version. Using the procedure reported by Shacham (1983), Dilorenzo et al. (1999) administered the POMS to a sample of breast cancer chemotherapy patients ($n$ = 114) and a sample of healthy adult women ($n$ = 55). Correlations between the long form and short form ranged between $r$ = .96 and $r$ = .99 for the six subscales in the healthy adult sample and between $r$ = .93 and $r$ = .99 for the breast cancer sample. The internal consistency of five of the six subscales was reported to be good to excellent for the breast cancer sample (coefficient alphas between .86 and .93) and excellent for the healthy adult sample (coefficient alphas between .90 and .97). The exception to this was the Confusion subscale in which coefficient alpha was .62 for the breast cancer sample and .73 for the healthy adult sample which was similar to the findings reported by Curran et al. (1995) for this particular subscale. Like Curran et al. (1995), DiLorenzo et al. (1999) concluded that the Shacham's (1983) short form version of the POMS is psychometrically sound and an alternative to the long form POMS.

Similar findings to those discussed above in relation to Shacham's (1983) short form POMS was reported by Baker et al. (2002). In a sample of 428 cancer patients, Baker et al. (2002) reported good to excellent internal consistency for five of the six subscales with coefficient alpha values ranging from .87 to .91. The internal consistency of the Confusion subscale was found to be adequate with a coefficient alpha value of .78 in this sample. Baker et al. (2002) also reported the first confirmatory factor analysis conducted on Shacham's (1983) short form POMS and concluded that the "... fit of the proposed model to the data is adequate" (p. 277).

Further support of Shacham's (1983) short form POMS was reported by Malouff, Schutte, and Ramerth (1985). Malouff et al. (1985) were interested in determining if the Depression subscale of the short form was psychometrically equivalent to the long form version of this particular subscale, and hence, they did not assess the other five identified subscales. Nonetheless, consistent with both Shacham's (1983) findings, and those of Curran et al. (1995), an excellent internal consistency coefficient alpha value of .94 was noted for this eight item subscale. Malouff et al. (1985) also found that this subscale demonstrated a strong positive correlation with a standardized depression measure and concluded that the short form Depression subscale was useful as a measure of depression when a very short and valid measure was needed.

As noted above, McNair et al. (1992) also created a shortened version of their long form POMS. This short form POMS is a 30 item version, which is seven items shorter than the Shacham (1983) version, and was created by removing psychometrically unsound items. Besides the obvious difference in the number of items on these two versions, it is important to note that there are differences in the items that comprise the McNair et al. (1992) short form version and Shacham's (1983) short form version.

In particular, Shacham's (1983) Depression scale includes eight adjectives, only two of which are in the McNair et al. (1992) version. Shacham's (1983) six item Vigor scale includes one additional adjective (*cheerful*) which is not in the McNair et al. (1992) scale. The five items in the Fatigue scales differ by two adjectives in the two short form versions. Shacham's (1983) Anger scale overlaps with McNair et al.'s (1992) for four of the five adjectives. Similarly, four of the five adjectives in the Tension scale appear on both versions of the short form POMS. Only three adjectives from McNair et al.'s (1992) Confusion scale overlaps with Shacham's (1983) scale.

McNair et al. (1992) reported acceptable reliability for their short form version but they did not examine the factorial structure of the short form. Most of the psychometric research on short form versions of the POMS has focused on Shacham's (1983) version, with very little attention directed to the McNair et al. (1992) short form version with the exception of two papers, as reviewed below.

Yeun and Shin-Park (2006) examined the internal consistency of the McNair et al. (1992) short form version in a sample of healthy American adults ($n$ = 69) and using a translated version of this instrument in a sample of healthy Korean adults ($n$ = 115). They reported adequate to good internal reliability values, based on coefficient alpha, in both samples for five of the six subscales. Specifically, for the American sample (Depression = .76, Vigor = .75, Tension = .82, Anger = .84, and Fatigue = .88) and for the Korean sample (Depression = .80, Vigor = .85, Tension = .83, Anger = .79, and Fatigue = .82). The coefficient alpha's for the Confusion subscale were somewhat lower in both samples (American sample = .71; Korean sample = .59). Similar internal reliability values for the McNair et al. (1992) short form POMS, based on coefficient alpha, were reported by Bourgeois et al. (2010). Alpha coefficients ranged from .67 to .90; more specifically, Depression = .83, Vigor = .89, Tension = .80, Anger = .86, and Confusion = .67, and Fatigue = .87.

Bourgeois et al. (2010) also conducted an exploratory factor analysis on the McNair et al. (1992) short form POMS. Utilizing a principal components factor analysis with promax rotation they reported a five factor solution based on eigenvalues (ev) greater than 1.0. The five factors were Vigor (ev = 10.46), Anger (ev = 3.45), Depression (ev = 1.76), Fatigue (ev = 1.55), and Tension (ev = 1.13).

Confusion, the hypothesized sixth factor, had an eigenvalue of .95 with three of the five items loading onto this factor (specifically, *bewildered, forgetful,* and *muddled* with respective factor loadings of .40, .37, and .34). The other two items, *efficient* and *confused*, that purportedly comprise the Confusion subscale loaded most highly on the Vigor (loading = .58) and Depression (loading = .35) subscales respectively. Based on these findings,

Bourgeois et al. (2010) concluded that strong support exists for at least five of the six factors.

It should be noted however, that in their study, Bourgeois et al. (2010) combined data from 15 separate projects conducted over a nine year period. More specifically, their sample consisted of a total of 1,760 participants ranging in age from 16 to 64 years and the data was obtained from classroom, laboratory, and field settings, the latter of which was collected just prior to a sporting competition.

Of the total sample, approximately 68% could be considered moderate to high level athletes with the remaining individuals in the sample consisting of undergraduate students. The present study was designed to further examine the factorial structure of the 30 item short form POMS (McNair et al.) in a healthy adult sample to assess if the six factor model, and corresponding scoring key, could be demonstrated.

# METHOD

## Participants, Materials and Procedure

Undergraduate participants ($N$ = 290; 122 men and 168 women) completed the short form POMS (McNair et al., 1992). The mean age for participants was 21.05 years ($SD$ = 3.9, range was 17 to 42).

# RESULTS

The Kaiser-Meyer-Olkin test was found to be .89 suggesting that the responses to the short form POMS (McNair et al., 1992) could be factor analyzed (Tabachnick and Fidell, 2001). Six factors were extracted based on visual examination of the scree plot, accounting for 60.37% of the variance.

A principal components analysis with VARIMAX rotation was then conducted. Table 1 lists the rotated factor structure with the adjectives grouped for their corresponding scale. Listed below is an analysis of the factors in terms of the factor plot as well as the internal consistency (coefficient alpha) values.

**Table 1. Factor Structure of the Short Form POMS**

| Adjective | Depression | Vigor | Fatigue | Anger | Tension | Confusion |
|---|---|---|---|---|---|---|
| Sad | **.60** | -.23 | -.26 | .20 | .10 | -.06 |
| Unworthy | **.60** | .02 | .14 | .17 | .02 | -.14 |
| *Discouraged* | .31 | -.19 | .16 | .14 | .25 | .31 |
| Lonely | **.67** | -.29 | -.09 | .04 | -.04 | .14 |
| Gloomy | **.54** | -.06 | .03 | .21 | .21 | -.08 |
| Lively | .09 | **.76** | -.13 | .02 | -.14 | .12 |
| Active | -.17 | **.79** | -.09 | -.06 | .18 | -.09 |
| Energetic | -.06 | **.86** | -.09 | .01 | .01 | .05 |
| Full of pep | .09 | **.82** | -.09 | -.02 | -.14 | -.01 |
| Vigorous | -.01 | **.80** | -.01 | .06 | .02 | -.08 |
| Worn out | -.08 | -.22 | **.74** | .04 | .12 | -.04 |
| Fatigued | -.14 | -.08 | **.87** | -.02 | .06 | -.08 |
| Exhausted | -.01 | -.11 | **.84** | -.01 | .07 | .07 |
| Sluggish | .23 | -.04 | **.73** | .06 | -.15 | .02 |
| Weary | .19 | .01 | **.59** | .10 | .07 | .02 |
| Angry | -.10 | -.01 | -.06 | **.84** | .03 | -.04 |
| Grouchy | -.01 | -.06 | .09 | **.78** | -.03 | -.04 |
| Annoyed | -.08 | -.05 | .04 | **.71** | .06 | .18 |
| Furious | .14 | .17 | .10 | **.64** | -.04 | -.12 |
| Bad-tempered | .08 | .04 | -.07 | **.73** | .02 | .10 |
| Tense | -.10 | -.18 | .05 | .19 | **.64** | .12 |
| *Shaky* | **.52** | .13 | .23 | .04 | .05 | .14 |
| Uneasy | .23 | .08 | .04 | .15 | **.56** | -.30 |
| Nervous | .12 | -.02 | -.04 | -.10 | **.80** | -.01 |
| Anxious | -.02 | .08 | .09 | -.01 | **.70** | .11 |
| *Confused* | **.59** | .11 | .05 | -.16 | .16 | .12 |
| *Muddled* | **.65** | .12 | .21 | .05 | .01 | -.03 |
| *Bewildered* | **.53** | .16 | .21 | .05 | .17 | -.13 |
| Efficient | -.01 | .04 | -.05 | .05 | .08 | **.84** |
| *Forgetful* | .26 | .18 | .16 | .16 | -.03 | .22 |

Factor loadings >.50 are in bold. Adjectives written in italics suggest the adjective does not load well onto its designated factor.

## Depression Factor

This factor was fairly well defined with the exception of the adjective *discouraged*, which was found to load onto the Depression and Confusion factors. The coefficient alpha value for the five item scale was .76, suggesting that the adjective *discouraged* could remain in the scale.

### Vigor, Fatigue, and Anger Factors

These factors were well defined in that the adjectives were found to load onto their designated factors. The coefficient alpha values for the Vigor, Fatigue, and Anger scales were .89, .87, and .80, respectively.

### Tension Factor

This factor was fairly well defined with the exception of the adjective *shaky*, which loaded onto the depression factor. The coefficient alpha value for the five items scale was .72, suggesting that the adjective *shaky* might be included in a total score calculation.

### Confusion Factor

This factor was not well defined. Three of the five adjectives loaded onto the depression factor and the adjective *forgetful*, did not load substantially onto any of the six factors. Only the marker adjective, *efficient* defined the confusion factor (which represents a bipolar marker for this scale). The reliability analysis suggested that the adjective *efficient*, if deleted from the other four adjectives would increase the coefficient alpha from .63 to .70, although the factor loadings found in the present study questions the measurement soundness of combining the remaining four adjectives in a total scale score.

## CONCLUSION

As discussed throughout this chapter, a great deal of research has been conducted over the years which have utilized various versions of the POMS questionnaire (McNair et al., 1992). The popularity of short form versions of this measurement instrument has increased primarily because of the shorter time period required for administration. However, very little research has been conducted that has directly examined the psychometric properties and factorial structure of McNair et al.'s (1992) short form version. As Bourgeois et al. (2010) state, "a psychometrically sound abbreviated version should be superior to the original POMS in most research applications" (p. 370). The findings presented herein examined the factorial structure of McNair et al.'s (1992) short form version of the POMS in an undergraduate sample. In general, the present findings converge with those reported by Bourgeois et al. (2010) and Yeun and Shin-Park (2006).

In terms of the internal reliability, the present study demonstrated acceptable to good coefficient alpha values for five of the six subscales ranging from .72 (Tension subscale) to .89 (Vigor subscale). These values are in line with those reported by Bourgeois et al. (2010) and Yeun and Shin-Park (2006). Similarly, the Confusion subscale in the present study had the lowest coefficient alpha value which converges with the two previously mentioned studies. As noted by Yeun and Shin-Park (2006) in relation to the Confusion subscale, there "is doubt as to whether the factor is a trait of cognitive inefficiency, a mood state, or both" (p. 1179). Regardless, it is clear that further refinement of the items on the Confusion subscale needs to be conducted especially as only one of the five adjectives for this dimension actually creates a separate factor, and that the adjective, *efficient*, on face value, does not seem to assess into a confused mood state.

The factor loadings for five of the six scales were good to excellent. The Vigor, Fatigue, and Anger factors all had excellent factor loadings in that their corresponding adjectives loaded highly together and onto only one factor (demonstrating simple structure). Two of the factors, Depression and Tension, showed good factor structure in that four of the five adjectives loaded together and defined their factors. For the Depression factor, the adjective *discouraged* cross-loaded with the sixth factor, Confusion (although this latter factor was poorly defined in terms of the factor loadings as only one marker adjective actually loaded onto the factor). For the Tension factor, the adjective *shaky* loaded higher onto the Depression factor. Possibly the participants in the present study had difficulty with the meaning of this adjective as is also had a loading onto the Depression factor of similar magnitude to four of the five Depression adjectives (and for the three Confusion adjectives: *confused*, *muddled*, and *bewildered*).

Although the present results need to be replicated in other samples, the results suggest that the Confusion dimension is poorly defined. Possibly this dimension should be removed from the scale as only one of the adjectives (*efficient*) defined the sixth factor, and as the adjective might suggest, the scale possibly should not be labelled as Confusion. One area of future research is to assess the groupings of the adjectives, possibly by using card sort techniques. If people are asked to group the adjectives into six conceptually related piles, it would be interesting to assess how these groups of adjectives compare to those in the proposed structure of the scale. In particular, do the adjectives which showed poor factor loadings in the present study appear in different piles by the card sorters? These answers are essential for better understanding the mood adjectives and how these terms are interpreted by individuals, as, as reviewed above, mood states are assessed in multiple areas and with various groups of people.

In conclusion, the present results suggest that five (Depression, Vigor, Fatigue, Anger, and Tension) of the six short form POMS dimensions created by McNair et al. (1992) demonstrate good internal consistency (coefficient alpha) values. These five scales also have good to excellent factor structure results. Caution is suggested for researchers and clinicians using the Confusion scale. It is suggested, based on the results of the present study, that individuals using this scale first establish the internal consistency (coefficient alpha) value of the items, before deciding if a scale score total should be computed and interpreted.

## REFERENCES

Aroian, K. J., Kulwicki, A., Kaskiri, E. A., Templin, T. N., and Wells, C. L. (2007). Psychometric evaluation of the Arabic language version of the Profile of Mood States. *Research in Nursing and Health, 30,* 531-541.

Baker, F., Denniston, M., Zabora, J., Polland, A., and Dudley, W. N. (2002). A POMS short form for cancer patients: Psychometric and structural evaluation. *Psych-Oncology, 11,* 273-281.

Berger, B. G., and Motl, R. W. (2000). Exercise and mood: A selective review and synthesis of research employing the Profile of Mood States. *Journal of Applied Sport Psychology, 12,* 69-92.

Bourgeois, A., LeUnes, A., and Meyers, M. (2010) Full-scale ad short-form of the Profile of Mood States: A factor analytic comparison. *Journal of Sport Behaviour, 33 (4),* 355-376.

Boyle, G. J. (1987). A cross validation of the factor structure of the Profile of Modd States: Were the factors correctly identified in the first instance. *Psychological Reports, 60,* 343-354.

Boyle, G. J. (1988). Central clinical states: An examination of the Profile of Mood States and the Eight State Questionnaire. *Journal of Psychopathology and Behavioral Assessment, 10 (3),* 205-215.

Curran, S. L., Andrykowski, M. A., and Studts, J. L. (1995). Short form of the Profile of Mood States (POMS-SF): Psychometric information. *Psychological Assessment, 7,* 80-83.

DiLorenzo, T. A., Bovbjerg, D. H., Montgomery, G. H., Valdimarsdottir, H., and Jacobsen, P. B. (1999). The application of a shortened version of the Profile of Mood States in a sample of breast cancer chemotherapy patients. *British Journal of Health Psychology, 4,* 315-325.

Dipietro, J. A., Costigan, K. A., and Sipsma, H. L. (2008). Continuity in self-report measures of maternal anxiety, stress, and depressive symptoms from pregnancy through two years postpartum. *Journal of Psychosomatic Obstetrics and Gynecology, 29 (2),* 115-124.

Fink, A. M., Eckhardt, A. L., Fennessy, M. M., Jones, J., Kruse, D., VanderZwan, K. J., Ryan, C. J., and Zerwic, J. J. (2010). Psychometric properties of three instruments to measure fatigue with myocardial infarction. *Western Journal of Nursing Research, 32 (7),* 967-983.

Gibson, S. J. (1997). The measurement of mood states in older adults. *Journal of Gerontology, 52B (4),* 167-174.

Grove, J. R., and Prapavessis, H. (1992). Preliminary evidence for the reliability and validity of an Abbreviated Profile of Mood States. *International Journal of Sport Psychology, 23,* 93-109.

Guadagnoli, E., and Mor, V. (1989). Measuring cancer patients' affect: Revisions and psychometric properties of the Profile of Mood States (POMS). *Psychological Assessment, 1 (2),* 150-154.

Hainer, B. L., and Palesch, Y. (1998). Symptoms of depression in residents: A South Carolina family practice research consortium study. *Academic Medicine, 73 (12),* 1305-1310.

Hill, C. M., and Hill, D. W. (1991). Influence of time of day on responses to the Profile of Mood States. *Perceptual and Motor Skills, 72,* 434.

Jacobson, A. F., Weiss, B. L., Steinbook, R. M., Brauzer, B., and Goldstein, B. J. (1978). The measurement of psychological states by use of factors derived from a combination of items from mood and symptom checklists. *Journal of Clinical Psychology, 34 (3),* 677-685.

Kaye, J. M., Lawton, M. P., Gitlin, L. N., Kleban, M. H., Windsor, L. A., and Kaye, D. (1988). Older people's performance on the Profile of Mood States (POMS). *Clinical Gerontologist, 7 (3/4),* 35-56.

LeUnes, A. (2000). Updated bibliography on the Profile of Mood States in sport and exercise psychology. *Journal of Applied Sport Psychology, 12,* 110-113.

LeUnes, A., and Burger, J. (1998). Bibliography on the Profile of Mood States in sport and exercise. *Journal of Sport Behavior, 21,* 53-70.

Malouff, J. M., Schutte, N. S., and Ramerth, W. (1985). Evaluation of a short form of the POMS-Depression scale. *Journal of Clinical Psychology, 41 (3),* 389-391.

McMahon, R. C., and Davidson, R. S. (1986). Concurrent validity of the clinical symptom syndrome scales of the Millon Clinical Multiaxial Inventory. *Journal of Clinical Psychology, 42 (6),* 908-912.

McNair, D. M., Heuchert, J. P., and Shilony, E. (2003). *Profile of Mood States: Bibliography 1964-2002.* Toronto, Ontario: Multi-Health Systems.

McNair, D. M., Lorr, M., and Droppleman, L. F. (1971). *Manual for the Profile of Mood States.* San Diego, CA: Educational and Industrial Testing Service.

McNair, D. M., Lorr, M., and Droppleman, L. F. (1992). *EdITS Manual for the Profile of Mood States.* San Diego, CA: EdITS Educational and Industrial Testing Service.

Meek, P. M., Nail, L. M., Barsevick, A., Schwartz, A. L., Stephen, S., Whitmer, K., Beck, S. L., Jones, L. S., and Walker, B. L. (2000). Psychometric testing of fatigue instruments for use with cancer patients. *Nursing Research, 49 (4),* 181-190.

Miller, B. P., and Edgington, G. P. (1984). Psychological mood state distortion in a sporting context. *Journal of Sport Behavior, 7 (3),* 91-94.

Norcross, J. C., Guadagnoli, E., and Prochaska, J. G. (1984). Factor structure of the Profile of Mood States (POMS): Two partial replications. *Journal of Clinical Psychology, 40 (5),* 1270-1277.

Patterson, K., Young, C., Woods, S. P., Vigil, O., Grant, I., Atkinson, J. H., and The HIV Neurobehavioral Research Center Group. (2006). Screening for major depression in persons with HIV infection: The concurrent predictive validity of the Profile of Mood States Depression-Dejection scale. *International Journal of Methods in Psychiatric Research, 15 (2),* 75-82.

Reddon, J. R., Marceau, R., and Holden, R. R. (1985). A confirmatory evaluation of the Profile of Mood States: Convergent and discriminant item validity. *Journal of Psychopathology and Behavioral Assessment, 7 (3),* 243-259.

Shacham, S. (1983). A shortened version of the Profile of Mood States. *Journal of Personality Assessment, 47,* 305-306.

Tabachnick, B. G. and Fidell, L. S. (2001). *Using multivariate statistics (4th edition).* Boston, MA: Allyn and Bacon.

Terry, P. C., Keohane, L., and Lane, H. (1996). Development and validation of a shortened version of the Profile of Mood States suitable for use with young athletes [Abstract]. *Journal of Sport Sciences, 14,* 49.

Tunis, S. L., Golbus, M. S., Copeland, K. L., Fine, B. A., Rosinsky, B. J., and Seely, L. (1990). Normative scores and factor structure of the Profile of Mood States for women seeking prenatal diagnosis for advanced maternal age. *Educational and Psychological Measurement, 50,* 309-324.

Watson, D. and Clark, L. A. (1997). Measurement and mismeasurement of mood: Recurrent and emergent issues. *Journal of Personality Assessment, 68 (2),* 267-296.

Wyrwich, K. W., and Yu, H. (2011). Validation of POMS questionnaire in postmenopausal women. *Quality of Life Research, 20,* 1111-1121.

Yeun, E. J., and Shin-Park, K. K. (2006). Verification of the Profile of Mood States-Brief: Cross-cultural analysis. *Journal of Clinical Psychology, 62,* 1173-1180.

In: Screening Tests
Editor: Marguerite Gauthier

ISBN: 978-1-62417-963-1
© 2013 Nova Science Publishers, Inc.

*Chapter 5*

# THE AUDIO RECORDED COGNITIVE SCREEN (ARCS): A FLEXIBLE AND VERSATILE INSTRUMENT FOR CLINIC OR RESEARCH

***Peter W. Schofield[1,2,*], Jeannette Lechner-Scott[3], Carmel Loughland[2] and Tammie Moore[1]***

[1]Neuropsychiatry Service, Hunter New England Mental Health, Newcastle, Australia

[2]Centre for Translational Neuroscience and Mental Health (CTNMH), Hunter New England Mental Health and the University of Newcastle, Australia

[3]Department of Medicine, John Hunter Hospital, Hunter Medical Research Institute (HMRI), Newcastle, Australia
Schizophrenia Research Institute (SRI), Sydney, Australia

## ABSTRACT

The ARCS was developed as a medium length cognitive battery that, by virtue of its novel means of administration, can also serve as a screening test. The ARCS includes tests of episodic verbal memory, verbal fluency, language (object naming), visuospatial ability, and attention/executive functioning that are administered via an audio device (e.g. MP3 player, CD player, computer). The patient (or study

* Corresponding author: Peter Schofield: Email: Peter.Schofield@hnehealth.nsw.gov.au.

participant) writes their responses to the questions in a booklet for later scoring. A preamble on the audio provides a clear and simple explanation as to how testing will be conducted. Testing lasts 34 minutes and is unsupervised. Patients who score 18/30 or more on the Mini Mental State Examination are typically able to complete testing with the ARCS.

The time-cost to the clinician for obtaining the results is minimal: about two minutes to set the patient up with the audio and response booklet and about 2-4 minutes for scoring into the accompanying excel spreadsheet scoring calculator. The calculator converts raw scores into demographically adjusted scores and also serves as a database. The current chapter reviews our experience with the ARCS, highlighting its flexibility, and discusses its potential use in a range of clinical and research settings.

## INTRODUCTION

There are many situations in which the results of a sensitive and specific cognitive assessment might be valuable as part of a comprehensive clinical assessment. Within elderly populations, cognitive decline due to a broad range of conditions is common. Younger individuals can also experience cognitive decline due to early onset neurodegenerative diseases or conditions such as traumatic brain injury, multiple sclerosis, or systemic lupus erythematosis [1-2].

In all cases, characterization of the cognitive syndrome, important both diagnostically and functionally, requires an objective cognitive assessment. However, limitations of clinicians' time and expertise in the administration of sensitive cognitive assessment instruments constitute well-recognised barriers to such an evaluation. With these concerns in mind, more than a decade ago we initiated a project to develop a cognitive instrument that would facilitate a relatively sophisticated appraisal of cognition at a time-cost to the clinician that is normally associated with brief cognitive screening. Other considerations that guided the instrument design included the following: 1) It should be able to function as a screening test, without important ceiling effects, such that good performance could responsibly be used to reassure the clinician and patient 2) It should probe the major cognitive domains and permit a graded characterization of performance within each domain 3) It should have a sound normative base taking due account of age, gender and education 4) It should take advantage of technology, but would be 'low tech' and not depend on computers for its administration. 5) It should be made widely available to clinicians who might value its unique properties.

Guided by these constraints, the Audio Recorded Cognitive Screen (ARCS) is a hybrid [3]. It can serve both as a screening test and a multi-domain graded assessment of cognition. It probes cognitive domains using, for the most part, conventional neuropsychological tests but also uses technology as a time and cost-saving device. Because the unsupervised patient responds to questions presented on an audio device by writing their answers in a specially designed booklet for later scoring, the raw data are preserved. Using a computer loaded with a customized excel 'ARCS calculator' program, demographically-adjusted scaled (domain-specific and overall) scores can be generated but a demographically-adjusted overall score can also be generated using simple arithmetic without the requirement for computer access [3]. We have established a website (www.cognitionhealth.com) through which the ARCS and all the material needed to administer and score it can be accessed by clinicians. We have opted to attach a relatively nominal cost to obtaining and using the ARCS to restrict its use to clinicians and to make access unappealing to lay individuals wishing to test themselves. We hoped thereby to avoid the potential risks associated with lay self-testing without professional input/review and protect the integrity of the instrument.

## ELEMENTS OF THE ARCS

With the first iteration of our test, which we called the Tape-Administered Cognitive Screen (TACS) [4], we explored the potential for administering cognitive tests via an audio device.

The Hopkins Verbal Learning Test –Revised (HVLT-R) [5] constituted the memory test in the TACS. Because it performed well we retained the overall structure of the HVLT-R but generated our own word lists, using the same strategy as described by Brandt [6], for the new memory test for the ARCS. Other modifications were made to the TACS to create the ARCS, the elements of which are outlined below.

The cognitive tests of the ARCS are administered via a simple audio device (CD player, MP3 player, or computer) to which the patient listens through headphones. The patient, who remains unsupervised throughout, responds to the tasks presented by writing in a specially designed response booklet, structured so as to facilitate the conduct of the testing even for quite impaired individuals (e.g. with Mini Mental State Scores (MMSE) [7] as low as 19). The ARCS comprises:

1) A 12-word list learning task, closely modelled on a well-validated 12 word list learning task, the HVLT-R [5]. Three learning trials are followed 20 minutes later by a free recall trial then a recognition trial.
2) A clock drawing task. Subjects are given 75 seconds to fill in the numbers around a pre-drawn circle to form a clock face, and draw the hands to indicate 10 past 11 [8].
3) Verbal fluency tasks. Subjects are given one minute each to write down words from a semantic category, action words (i.e. verbs), and words beginning with a particular letter.
4) Speed of writing test. Subjects are requested to write the word 'table' as many times as they can in 30 seconds.
5) Object naming. Subjects are requested to identify in writing the names of ten different objects depicted in the response booklet.
6) The 'Hunter Attentional Task' (HAT). This test has two parts. In part one (i.e. HAT A), the subject is presented with an array of letters, all written in lower case, and is required to write the same letter alongside each, but in upper case form. In part two (i.e. HAT B), the subject is presented with the same array of letters (again, all in lower case), but a pseudo-random 50% of the letters have been circled. The subject is required to write the same letter beside each letter -- in upper case after the non-circled letters, but in lower case after the circled letters -- in sequence, missing no letters across the page. For both parts, the subject has 30 seconds to copy as many letters as possible.

At the end of the audio and following completion of the cognitive tasks, patients respond to written questions included as a continuation of the response booklet. These questions request demographic information and self-rating of performance on the test and query any problems in the practical conduct of testing, as described later. The audio component of the ARCS lasts about 34 minutes, during which time the patient remains unsupervised. The results of the testing are obtained at the total time-cost to the clinician of the several minutes needed for set up and an additional 2-4 minutes necessary for scoring. Assistants can readily be trained to perform both these procedures. Two versions of the ARCS are available, differing in the memory test word-list and the semantic category and letter fluency tasks.

# Properties
## Scope and Normative Database

As outlined above, the ARCS probes the major cognitive domains relevant to a comprehensive cognitive assessment. Table 1 shows the results of a factor analysis conducted on 183 individuals who had undergone both the ARCS and a neuropsychological test battery [3].

**Table 1. Principal components analysis of raw ARCS measures and selected raw neuropsychological tests: 5 factors extracted (oblique rotation), accounting for 72.4% of the variance ($n$ = 183)**

| Measure | Component | | | | |
|---|---|---|---|---|---|
| | I | II | III | IV | V |
| | (Executive functioning/ attention) | (Memory) | (Verbal fluency) | (Language) | (Visuospatial) |
| Symbol Digit (written) | 0.83 | | | | |
| Trails B | -0.81 | | | | |
| Symbol Digit (oral) | 0.78 | | | | |
| Stroop inhibition | -0.77 | | | | |
| *ARCS: HAT B* | *0.57* | 0.30 | | | |
| Trails A | -0.52 | | | | -0.31 |
| RAVLT: | | | | | |
| Delayed recall (trial 7) | | 0.92 | | | |
| Discrimination index | | 0.88 | | | |
| Immediate recall (trials 1-5) | | 0.80 | | | |
| *ARCS - NAVLT:* | | | | | |
| *Delayed recall (trial 4)* | | *0.73* | | | |
| *Discrimination index* | | *0.71* | | | |
| *Immediate recall (trials 1-3)* | | *0.59* | | | |
| *ARCS: Letter Fluency* | | | *0.90* | | |
| CFL word fluency | | | 0.86 | | |
| *ARCS: Action fluency* | | | *0.67* | | |
| *ARCS: Category fluency* | | | *0.61* | | |
| Category fluency | | | 0.38 | | 0.34 |
| *ARCS: Object naming* | | | | *0.93* | |

**Table 1. (Continued)**

| Measure | Component | | | | |
|---|---|---|---|---|---|
| | I | II | III | IV | V |
| | (Executive functioning/ attention) | (Memory) | (Verbal fluency) | (Language) | (Visuospatial) |
| Boston Naming | | | | 0.74 | |
| Rey Complex Figure – copy | | | | | 0.66 |
| Block Design | 0.41 | | | | 0.50 |
| Visual Reproduction | | 0.30 | | | 0.47 |
| *ARCS: Clock drawing* | | | | | *0.41* |

All factor loadings above ±0.30 are reported. ARCS, Audio Recorded Cognitive Screen; CFL, measure of phonemic word fluency; HAT, Hunter Attentional Task; NAVLT, Newcastle Auditory Verbal Learning Test; RAVLT, Rey Auditory Verbal Learning Test.

The ARCS elements loaded onto five domains which we named memory, executive functioning/attention, language, (i.e. object naming), verbal fluency, and visuospatial functioning. Several domain scores are derived from the results from multiple tests. Our scoring program generates scaled scores—taking account of demographic norms—for individual tests as well as for the domain scores. Except for one of the component tests, all elements of the ARCS have a rich history. The exception is the Hunter Attentional Task (HAT), a test described above with two elements: HAT A and HAT B. As demonstrated in Table 1, the HAT B shares variance with well-recognised tests that are sensitive to executive dysfunction. Tests of verbal fluency, of which three are included in the ARCS, are also sensitive to 'frontal lobe' or executive dysfunction and in respect of its examination of this aspect of cognitive functioning, the ARCS compares favourably with many other cognitive screening instruments [9]. Normative scores that were used to define scaling paradigms were derived from the results of testing 550 community dwelling individuals ranging in age from 18-84 years. Scaled scores are generated from raw scores such that, for any single test, domain score, or indeed the overall score, a normal (scaled) score is 100 with a population standard deviation of 15. Using 1.5 standard deviations below normal to flag the possibility of decline implies that scores below 78 might appropriately attract some level of concern.

## VALIDITY

Validity of the ARCS has been examined in a variety of contexts and the results from these studies have been published elsewhere [3,10-11]. Individual elements of the ARCS correlate moderately to well with corresponding conventional neuropsychological tests (Table 2).

**Table 2. Correlations between raw ARCS measures and selected raw neuropsychological, tests ($n$ = 183)**

| ARCS domain | ARCS measure | Neuropsychological test | Correlation coefficient† |
|---|---|---|---|
| | | | |
| Memory | NAVLT:<br>Delayed recall (trial 4) | RAVLT:<br>Delayed recall (trial 7) | 0.69 |
| | Discrimination index | Discrimination index | 0.67 |
| | Immediate recall (trials 1-3) | Immediate recall (trials 1-5) | 0.66 |
| | Immediate recall | Visual Reproduction | 0.59 |
| Fluency | Letter | CFL word fluency | 0.69 |
| | Category | Category fluency | 0.51 |
| | Action | CFL word fluency | 0.50 |
| | | | |
| Visuospatial | Clock drawing | Visual Reproduction | 0.63 |
| | | Block Design | 0.56 |
| | | Rey Complex Figure - copy | 0.53 |
| | | | |
| Language | Object naming | Boston Naming | 0.70 |
| | | | |
| Attention | HAT B | Symbol Digit (written) | 0.68 |
| | | Symbol Digit (oral) | 0.64 |
| | | Stroop inhibition | -0.51 |
| | | Trails B | -0.47 |
| | | Trails A | -0.44 |

ARCS, Audio Recorded Cognitive Screen; CFL, measure of phonemic word fluency; HAT, Hunter Attentional Task; NAVLT, Newcastle Auditory Verbal Learning Test; RAVLT, Rey Auditory Verbal Learning Test. † All correlations are statistically significant (minimum $p$<0.001).

Total score on the ARCS has been shown, significantly better than the MMSE, to differentiate cognitively intact individuals from those with cognitive impairment and those with dementia from heterogeneous causes as determined by gold standard assessments.

Among individuals with multiple sclerosis, the ARCS was more sensitive than the Paced Auditory Serial Addition Test, (a screening instrument widely used for detection of cognitive changes in that disorder), in detecting cognitive impairment as independently determined by gold standard conventional neuropsychological testing [10]. In another study which compared the results of cognitive testing in controls and individuals with a psychotic illness (most due to schizophrenia) group-specific differences in ARCS scores were at least as great as those on the Repeatable Battery for the Assessment of Neuropsychological Status (RBANS), a conventional neuropsychological test battery that takes about 30 minutes to administer [12].

## RELIABILITY

We reported alternate form reliability in our first publication on the ARCS, with correlation coefficients ranging from 0.70 (HAT B) to 0.88 for the overall ARCS in a sample of 22 individuals for inter-test intervals from 24-168 days [3].

The two alternate forms of the ARCS have different memory word lists and letter and category fluency items but action fluency, clock drawing, the pictured items for naming and the HAT are common to both. In a more recent analysis of 105 individuals attending our neuropsychiatry outpatients who underwent a repeat (alternate form) ARCS within a year (mean 133 days, SD 78) – patients in whom both improvement and decline are potential clinical courses-- the correlations for repeat alternate form testing by cognitive domain were:

Memory 0.71, Fluency 0.81, Visuospatial 0.73, Language 0.77, Attention 0.60, Overall ARCS 0.84. Improvements in mean domain scores (paired t-tests) were seen for Memory (66.5 to 70.2, p=0.09), Visuospatial (90.7-93.8, p=0.039), Language (82.1-86.6, p=0.002) Attention (83.1-86.0, p=0.01) and Overall ARCS (68.7-73.5, p=0.00). Domains for which there are alternate forms did *not* show statistically significant improvement and the slight but statistically significant improvement in the domain elements common to both forms of the ARCS may reflect learning effects on repeat testing.

We assessed interscorer reliability in 20 randomly chosen booklets and found it to be high even for elements potentially subject to interpretation. Scoring templates assist scoring for the clock drawing task and the delayed recognition trial of the memory list learning task.

## SENSITIVITY AND SPECIFICITY

Close examination of normative data identified significant effects of gender, education and age on ARCS test performance and the paradigms by which we derive scaled scores is based on a relatively highly fractionated normal population with demographically-specific cells for each of four age categories, four education categories, and gender (i.e. 32 cells). A consequence of this approach has been to generate quite narrow normative ranges, particularly for younger and highly educated individuals. Accordingly, our scaled scores may flag the possibility of cognitive impairment at higher levels of performance than some comparator tests. In a study of 183 individuals comprising a clinic sample and a 'validation sample' of individuals shown to be free of cognitive impairment on the same battery of neuropsychological tests used to characterize the clinic sample, the overall ARCS showed good excellent sensitivity (92%) and specificity (90%) (Area under the Curve (AUC) 0.98) comparing very favourably with the Mini Mental State Examination (MMSE) (sensitivity 0.78, specificity 0.85, AUC 0.91) [3]. For the detection of cognitive impairment or dementia, the ARCS fared even better (sensitivity 0.83, specificity 0.82 AUC 0.90), relative to the MMSE (sensitivity 0.62, specificity 0.65, AUC 0.71). We are progressively collecting data in a wide range of contexts to facilitate the reporting of the psychometric properties for the detection of cognitive impairment or dementia due to diverse aetiologies.

## SPECIAL FEATURES

### 'Interface' Issues

Several novel features of the ARCS warrant particular attention as they have the potential to impact performance and the validity of testing. Because the test is administered unsupervised, there is no potential for the patient to seek clarification of instructions or repetition if a word is not clearly heard (for example on the list learning task). We sought to minimize problems by making instructions on the recording very simple and clear, with judicious repetition, so that individuals with memory impairment would not be penalized on tasks designed to probe non-memory cognitive domains. The male voice on the audio is pleasant to listen to and has a neutral accent. Once the test begins, the audio provides precisely defined intervals of time for responses to each cognitive task, an instance of the high level of standardization implicit in this mode of presentation. As far as we are aware, no other test developer has adopted our approach of administering test material by audio and requiring written responses. An advantage of this approach is that it simplifies the interface issue, relative, for example, to computer based tests (CBTs) as there is no requirement for training or initial supervision to establish that the mode of responding to questions has been mastered [13]. Many CBTs do not assess free recall of memory tasks either in learning or delayed recall trials [13], but these elements are part of the ARCS and replicate the structure of conventional list learning tasks such as the HVLT-R or the California Verbal Learning Test [14]. Also by contrast with many CBTs the ARCS probes verbal fluency and object naming, abilities routinely assessed in conventional neuropsychological testing.

By design, we provided what we considered to be ample time for most individuals to complete 'non-timed' tasks (memory, object naming, clock drawing) but we imposed time limits for the verbal fluency and the Hunter Attentional Tasks.

It is possible therefore that an individual's writing speed could impact their performance on the timed tasks or even, if very slow, on the 'untimed' tasks. Our cognitively non-challenging 'writing speed' task was included as an element that might be valuable, in individual cases, to flag such a possible confound. Because of the possible relevance of these issues for performance on the ARCS, we included the following written multiple choice questions at the end of the response booklet:

1) Could you hear the instructions on the recording clearly? (possible responses a) yes all the time b) occasionally I had difficulty hearing c) No, I had trouble hearing what was said most of the time).
2) Did you find the directions on the recording confusing or difficult to follow? (possible responses a) no, I understood the instructions clearly b) sometimes c) most of the time d) I cannot recall whether the instructions were easy or difficult to understand).

To explore the potential impact of these interface issues, we have conducted a series of hierarchical linear regression analyses within a sample of 121 clinic patients (70 (58%) males; mean age 56.1y range 18-87; mean overall ARCS 71.3, SD 24.6) who had had both the ARCS and a neuropsychological assessment administered within one year of each other (mean 109 days). We dichotomised responses to the question about hearing (could hear 'yes, all the time' (n=115, (95%)) vs the rest) and 'confusion?' ('understood the instructions clearly' (n=102, (84%)) vs the rest). For each analysis, the raw score of an ARCS test representative of one of the 5 cognitive domains was the dependent variable. We first entered age, gender and education (step 1) then the raw score of the appropriate corresponding conventional neuropsychological test (step 2), then sought the additional variance in ARCS raw score explained by writing speed (step 3), or hearing difficulties and confusion (step 4). Thus, for example, in a regression analysis predicting delayed free recall on the memory test of the ARCS, the variance (R Square ($R^2$)) explained by age, gender and education (step 1) was 0.162 $p<0.001$.

The incremental variance (i.e. $R^2$ change) explained by delayed free recall on the Rey Auditory Verbal Learning Test (RAVLT) (step 2) was 0.376, $p<0.001$), by writing speed (step 3) $R^2$ change was 0.001, $p=0.69$, and by hearing/confusion (Step 4) $R^2$ change was 0.04, $p<0.01$.

**Table 3. Results from 5 hierarchical linear regression analyses predicting raw ARCS test scores in 121 individuals. Cells show $R^2$ change and level of statistical significance**

| ARCS test / Step | Delayed recall | HAT B[1] | Letter Fluency | Clock drawing | Naming |
|---|---|---|---|---|---|
| 1.Age, gender Education | 0.162** | 0.158** | 0.121** | 0.060 | 0.017 |
| 2.Comparison Neuropsych test | 0.376** RAVLT[2] delayed recall | 0.114** SDOMT[3] | 0.333** Letter fluency | 0.182** Rey complex figure copy | 0.238** Boston Naming Test |
| 3.Writing Speed | 0.001 | 0.074** | 0.026* | 0.002 | 0.003 |
| 4.Hearing confusion | 0.037* | 0.035 | 0.015 | 0.013 | 0.081** |

1 Hunter Attentional Task B; 2.Rey Auditory Verbal Learning Test; 3.Symbol Digit Modality Test (oral version). *p<0.05, **p<0.01.

Overall, in these hierarchical regression analyses, the $R^2$ change explained by writing speed varied from 0.001 (p=0.696) for delayed memory to 0.07 (p=0.001) for HAT B, and the $R^2$ change for hearing/confusion ranged from 0.013 (p=0.383) for clock drawing to 0.081 (p=0.002) for object naming. In summary, although statistically significant in several instances, the interface factors of writing speed, hearing difficulties, and difficulty understanding instructions contributed relatively very little to the performance on key elements of the ARCS in this clinically heterogeneous sample of patients, which included many with significant levels of cognitive impairment.

### Potential for Cheating (Faking Good)

Because the ARCS is conducted unsupervised, there is the potential for test participants to look back at their previous answers (for example during the learning trials of the memory test) to enhance their performance. That is, by contrast with virtually all other cognitive assessment instruments, individuals can theoretically not only fake bad but also fake good. In clinical practice there are circumstances in which the clinician might anticipate that a patient might wish to fake good. (e.g. their capacity to drive is being questioned). In such cases, it would be prudent to avoid administering the ARCS or, as we have done on rare occasions, have someone sit in on the assessment to observe the patient's behaviour during testing.

## Practical Aspects

### Administration

Testing is best conducted in a quiet room at a table with the patient facing away from the door in case someone inadvertently opens the door during testing. It is important to check that the patient is confident that they will not need to use the bathroom for at least 40 minutes, and that any mobile phone is turned off or onto' silent' for the duration of testing. The audio on the ARCS begins with a gentle preamble that explains to the patient how the testing will proceed. Accordingly, the clinician does not need to prepare the patient for testing with detailed explanations. However it is important to check that the patient is able to write and if this has not already been established it is achieved, albeit in limited fashion, by having the patient write their name and the date of testing on the front cover of the response booklet. To check on the patient's capacity to read, and that visual acuity is adequate for testing, patients are instructed to read the following sentence, printed in relative small type on the front cover of the response booklet: 'If you have reading glasses you should put them on now to do this assessment'. Once the audio is commenced, it is important that the volume is adjusted to an adequate level as determined by feedback from the patient.

### Scoring: QuickARCS and Computer-Based Scaling

The most comprehensive and detailed demographically adjusted (scaled) scores of individual tests, cognitive domains and overall (global) score are obtained by entering raw test scores into an excel spreadsheet calculator program which also serves as an accumulating database from which previously entered scores can be readily retrieved (see www.cognitionhealth.com). At the time of testing, patients record their age, gender, and educational attainment at the back of the response booklet and scoring can be done at any time after testing by a suitably trained tester who has familiarized themselves with the scoring routines from the scoring manual. Once familiar with the routines, scoring takes about two minutes. Clinicians lacking access to a computer can compute a demographically adjusted overall score on the ARCS by a simple arithmetic combination of key ARCS test raw scores and the addition of a unique correction factor, read from a simple table, which is determined by the patient's age, gender and education [3].

## Current Experience and Potential Uses

Our greatest experience with the ARCS has been in the context of specialty (neuropsychiatry, memory disorders, and multiple sclerosis) outpatient clinics where it functions particularly well as part of an initial intensive assessment. While the patient undergoes the unsupervised testing with the ARCS, more detailed history can be taken from an informant. Because scoring is achieved very efficiently, the results are available by the end of the consultation to help guide subsequent management. We use the results to identify individuals who would most benefit from further detailed neuropsychological assessment, those who can be reassured because they perform well, and those who may warrant repeated testing with the ARCS in a year or so. Results generated by the scoring program may characterize a pattern of cognitive impairment that is useful both diagnostically and in determining a patient's current cognitive strengths and weaknesses. And, in the context of the multiple sclerosis clinic in particular, the ARCS has been very valuable as a means of tracking cognitive change. As with any cognitive test, the results of the ARCS need to be interpreted within the larger context of the patient's history, the findings on examination and, if appropriate, additional investigations.

Within a primary care setting, the ARCS has the potential to help decide who should be referred for specialist evaluation. Because the ARCS has high sensitivity and a broad normative base across the full adult age range, good performance on the test provides the clinician with grounds for reassuring the patient. Highly educated individuals with cognitive concerns who score well on a screening instrument such as the MMSE, for example, currently present a challenge to the primary care clinician. The ARCS may provide valuable clarification under such circumstances.

We have used the ARCS as an efficient means of characterizing cognition in clinic-based research settings but the ARCS is also the principal cognitive assessment instrument used in a large community-based longitudinal study of aging in the Hunter Region of New South Wales [15-16]. In both settings, the minimal need for resources required to obtain the results of testing constitute a major advantage.

## ACKNOWLEDGMENTS

We would like to thank all the participants in our studies for their time and cooperation.

Tables 1 and 2 are reprinted from Schofield et al. J Neurol Neurosurg Psychiatry 2010; 2010, 81, 605 with permission.

## REFERENCES

[1] Schofield, P. Dementia associated with toxic causes and autoimmune disease. *International Psychogeriatrics,* 2005, Suppl 1, S129-147.

[2] McMurtray, A; Clark, DG; Christine, D; Mendez, MF. Early-onset dementia: frequency and causes compared to late-onset dementia. *Dementia and Geriatric Cognitive Disorders,* 2006, 21, 59-64.

[3] Schofield, PW; Lee, SJ; Lewin, TJ; Lyall, G; Moyle, J; Attia, J; McEvoy, M. The Audio Recorded Cognitive Screen (ARCS): a flexible hybrid cognitive test instrument. Journal of Neurology, *Neurosurgery and Psychiatry,* 2010, 81, 602-607.

[4] Schofield, PW; Lee, SJ; Davies, GC. Cognitive screening using a tape recorder: a pilot study. *Journal of the American Geriatrics Society,* 2003, 3, 415-418.

[5] Benedict, RHB; Schretlen, D; Groninger, L; Brandt, J. Hopkins Verbal Learning Test-Revised: Normative Data and analysis of inter-form and test-retest reliability. *Clinical Neuropsychology,* 1998, 12, 43-55.

[6] Brandt, J. The Hopkins Verbal Learning Test: development of a new memory test with six equivalent forms. *Clinical Neuropsychology,* 1991, 5, 125-142.

[7] Folstein, MF; Folstein, SE; McHugh, PR. Mini-Mental State: a practical method for grading the cognitive state of patients for the clinician. *Journal of Psychiatric Research,* 1975, 12, 189-198.

[8] Manos, PJ; Wu, R. The ten point clock test: a quick screen and grading method for cognitive impairment in medical and surgical patients. *International Journal of Psychological Medicine,* 1994, 24, 229-244.

[9] Cullen B, O'Neill B, Evans JJ, Coen RF, Lawlor BA. A review of screening tests for cognitive impairment. *Journal of Neurology Neurosurgery and Psychiatry,* 2007,78,790-799.

[10] Lechner-Scott, J; Kerr, T; Spencer, B; Agland, S; Lyndon, A; Schofield, PW. The Audio recorded Cognitive Screen (ARCS) in patients with multiple Sclerosis: a practical tool for multiple sclerosis clinics. *Multiple Sclerosis,* 2010, 16, 1126-1133.

[11] Loughland CM; Allen, J; Gianacas, L; Schofield, PW; Lewin, TJ; Hunter, M; Carr, VJ. Brief neuropsychological profiles in psychosis: a pilot study using the Audio Recorded Cognitive Screen (ARCS). *Acta. Neuropsychiatrica,* 2010, 22, 243-252.

[12] Gold JM, Queern C, Iannone VN, Buchanan RW. Repeatable Battery for the Assessment of Neuropsychological Status as a screening test in schizophrenia, I: sensitivity, reliability and validity. *American Journal of Psychiatry,* 1999, 156, 1944–1950.

[13] Wild, K; Howieson, D; Webbe, F; Seelye, A; Kaye, J. Status of computerized cognitive testing in aging: a systematic review. *Alzheimer's and Dementia,* 2008, 4, 428-437.

[14] Delis, DC; Kramer, JH; Kaplan, E; and Ober, BA. California Verbal Learning Test – Second Edition, Adult Version. San Antonio, Texas: The Psychological Corporation; 2000.

[15] Schofield, PW; Ebrahimi, H; Jones, AE; Bateman, GA; Murray, SR. An olfactory 'stress test' may detect preclinical Alzheimer's disease. *BMC Neurology,* 2012, 12, 24-31.

[16] McEvoy, M; Smith, W; D'Este, C; Duke, J; Peel, R; Schofield, PW; Scott, R; Byles, J; Henry, D; Ewald, B; Hancock, S; Smith, D; Attia, J. Cohort profile: The hunter community study. *International Journal of Epidemiology,* 2010, 39, 1452-1463.

# INDEX

## A



## B

## C

## D



## E

## L



## M

## Q



## R

U



V



W



X



Y